HEALTH CARE IN THE UNITED STATES: DEVELOPMENTS AND CONSIDERATIONS

HEALTH CARE IN THE UNITED STATES

DEVELOPMENTS AND CONSIDERATIONS

VOLUME 2

HEALTH CARE IN THE UNITED STATES: DEVELOPMENTS AND CONSIDERATIONS

Additional books in this series can be found on Nova's website under the Series tab.

Additional E-books in this series can be found on Nova's website under the E-book tab.

HEALTH CARE IN THE UNITED STATES:
DEVELOPMENTS AND CONSIDERATIONS

HEALTH CARE IN THE UNITED STATES

DEVELOPMENTS AND CONSIDERATIONS

VOLUME 2

LEONE GIANGIULIO
EDITOR

nova publishers
New York

For permission to use material from this book please contact us:
Telephone 631-231-7269; Fax 631-231-8175
Web Site: http://www.novapublishers.com

Library of Congress Cataloging-in-Publication Data

ISBN: 978-1-62618-413-8
ISSN: 2325-632X

Published by Nova Science Publishers, Inc. † New York

CONTENTS

PREFACE

The health care reform debate in the United States raises many complex issues including those of coverage, accessibility, cost, accountability, and quality of health care. Underlying these policy considerations are issues regarding the status of health care as a constitutional or legal right. This book series analyzes the constitutional and legal issues pertaining to the right of health care and the power of Congress to enact and fund health care programs. Other topics discussed in this volume include health care price transparency; private health insurance and estimates of individuals with pre-existing conditions which range from 36 million to 122 million; expiration of the health coverage tax credit and how it will affect participants' costs and coverage choices as health reform provisions are implemented; trends, vulnerabilities and recommendations in personal care services; and traditional versus benchmark benefits under medicaid.

Chapter 1 – In recent years, consumers have become responsible for a growing proportion of the costs of their health care. Health care price information that is transparent—available before consumers receive care—may help consumers anticipate these costs. Research identifies meaningful types of health care price information, such as estimates of what the complete cost will be to the consumer for a service. GAO defines an estimate of a consumer's complete health care cost as price information on a service that identifies a consumer's out-of-pocket cost, including any negotiated discounts, and all costs associated with a service or services. GAO examined (1) how various factors affect the availability of health care price information for consumers and (2) the information selected public and private health care price transparency initiatives make available to consumers. To do this work, GAO reviewed price transparency literature; interviewed experts; and examined a total of eight selected federal, state, and private insurance company health care price transparency initiatives. In addition, GAO anonymously contacted providers and requested the price of selected services to gain a consumer's perspective.

Chapter 2 – Individuals who buy coverage directly from a health insurer are often denied coverage due to a pre-existing condition during a process called medical underwriting, which assesses an applicant's health status and other risk factors. Beginning January 1, 2014, the Patient Protection and Affordable Care Act (PPACA) prohibits health insurers in the individual market from denying coverage, increasing premiums, or restricting benefits because of a pre-existing condition. GAO was asked to examine the effect of this provision on adults who are 19- 64 years old. GAO examined (1) the most common medical conditions that would cause an insurance company to restrict or deny insurance coverage for adults and the average annual costs associated with these conditions, (2) estimates of the number of adults with pre-existing conditions, and (3) the geographic and demographic profile of adults with pre-existing conditions.

To address these three issues, GAO (1) identified four recent studies that narrowly or more broadly identified five lists of conditions likely to result in restricted coverage in the individual insurance market and (2) used the 2009 Medical Expenditure Panel Survey to generate five separate estimates, referred to as estimates 1 through 5. There is no commonly accepted list of pre-existing conditions because each insurer determines the conditions it will use for medical underwriting. The authors also contacted state insurance department officials in all 50 states and the District of Columbia to confirm information about state insurance protections that currently limit or prohibit medical underwriting.

Chapter 3 – The HCTC pays 72.5 percent of health plan premiums for certain workers who lost their jobs due to foreign import competition and for certain retirees whose pensions from their former employers were terminated and are now paid by the Pension Benefit Guaranty Corporation. A small share of individuals who are potentially eligible for the HCTC participate. In 2010 there were 43,864 participants and 469,168 nonparticipants. The HCTC program will expire at the end of 2013 when premium tax credits and cost-sharing subsidies become available to eligible individuals who purchase health plans through health insurance exchanges under PPACA. PPACA also expands Medicaid eligibility to nonelderly individuals who meet specific income requirements to the extent that states choose to implement this provision. Therefore, the costs for health plans and coverage available to individuals potentially eligible for the HCTC will change when the HCTC expires.

This report examines (1) how the HCTC's expiration and the implementation of the PPACA premium tax credit, cost-sharing subsidies, and Medicaid expansion will affect HCTC participants and nonparticipants, and (2) how the coverage that will be available through the PPACA exchanges compares to HCTC participants' health plan coverage. GAO analyzed 2010 HCTC program data and individual tax filer data. GAO also compared the services and actuarial values of the plans that will be available through the exchanges to HCTC plans.

Chapter 4 – The Office of Inspector General's (OIG) body of work examining Medicaid personal care services (PCS) has found significant and persistent compliance, payment, and fraud vulnerabilities that demonstrate the need for Centers for Medicare & Medicaid Services (CMS) to take a more active role with States to combat these issues.

In 2011, Medicaid costs for PCS totaled approximately $12.7 billion, a 35-percent increase since 2005. Several Federal court decisions and Department of Health and Human Services policy initiatives aimed at providing more home and community-based options to Medicaid beneficiaries contribute to the increase in PCS use. As more and more State Medicaid programs explore home care options like PCS, it is critical that adequate safeguards exist to prevent fraud, waste, and abuse in PCS and other important home care benefits.

This document summarizes OIG's PCS work and, on the basis of the analysis of this work in the aggregate, offers recommendations to improve the integrity of Medicaid PCS.

Chapter 5 – The Medicaid program, which served 69 million people in FY2011, finances the delivery of a wide variety of preventive, primary and acute care services as well as long-term services and supports for certain low-income populations. Benefits are available to beneficiaries through two avenues. First, the traditional Medicaid program covers a wide variety of mandatory services (e.g., inpatient hospital services, lab/x-ray services, physician care, nursing facility care for persons aged 21 and over) and other services at state option (e.g., prescribed drugs, physician-directed clinic services, physical therapy, prosthetic devices) to the majority of Medicaid beneficiaries across the United States. Within broad federal guidelines, states define the amount, duration, and scope of these benefits. Thus, even mandatory services are not identical from stateto-state.

The Deficit Reduction Act of 2005 (DRA; P.L. 109-171) created an alternative benefit structure for Medicaid. Under this authority, states may enroll certain Medicaid subpopulations into benchmark benefit plans that include four choices: (1) the standard Blue Cross/Blue Shield preferred provider plan under the Federal Employees Health Benefits Program, (2) a plan offered to state employees, (3) the largest commercial health maintenance organization in the state, and (4) other coverage appropriate for the targeted population, subject to approval by the Secretary of Health and Human Services (HHS).

Since the enactment of the Patient Protection and Affordable Care Act in 2010 (ACA; P.L. 111- 148, as amended), benchmark benefits have taken on a new importance in the Medicaid program. As per the ACA, a new mandatory group of non-elderly, non-pregnant adults with income up to 133% of the federal poverty level will be eligible for Medicaid beginning in 2014, or sooner at state option. These individuals will be required to enroll in benchmark plans rather than traditional Medicaid (with some exceptions for subgroups with special medical needs). However, to date, only a handful of states have experience administering these plans, nearly all of which have been tailored to specific subpopulations.

The Congressional Budget Office (CBO) and the Joint Committee on Taxation (JCT) estimated that coverage expansion provisions in the ACA would increase enrollment by about 7 million in FY2014, rising to 11 million by FY2022 in both the Medicaid and the State Children's Health Insurance Programs (Congressional Budget Office, Estimates for the Insurance Coverage Provisions of the Affordable Care Act Updated for the Recent Supreme Court Decision, July 2012). Many of these new enrollees will get benchmark benefits. To assist Congress in evaluating the current scope of benefits available under Medicaid, this report outlines the major rules that govern and define both traditional Medicaid and benchmark benefits. It also compares the similarities and differences between these two benefit package designs.

In: Health Care in the United States
Editor: Leone Giangiulio
ISBN: 978-1-62618-413-8

Chapter 1

Health Care Price Transparency: Meaningful Price Information Is Difficult for Consumers to Obtain Prior to Receiving Care*

United States Government Accountability Office

Why GAO Did This Study

In recent years, consumers have become responsible for a growing proportion of the costs of their health care. Health care price information that is transparent—available before consumers receive care—may help consumers anticipate these costs. Research identifies meaningful types of health care price information, such as estimates of what the complete cost will be to the consumer for a service. GAO defines an estimate of a consumer's complete health care cost as price information on a service that identifies a consumer's out-of-pocket cost, including any negotiated discounts, and all costs associated with a service or services. GAO examined (1) how various factors affect the availability of health care price information for consumers and (2) the information selected public and private health care price transparency initiatives make available to consumers. To do this work, GAO reviewed price

* This is an edited, reformatted and augmented version of United States Government Accountability Office, Publication No. GAO-11-791, dated September 2011.

transparency literature; interviewed experts; and examined a total of eight selected federal, state, and private insurance company health care price transparency initiatives. In addition, GAO anonymously contacted providers and requested the price of selected services to gain a consumer's perspective.

What GAO Recommends

GAO recommends that the Department of Health and Human Services (HHS) determine the feasibility of making estimates of complete costs of health care services available to consumers, and, as appropriate, identify next steps. HHS reviewed a draft of this report and provided technical comments, which GAO incorporated as appropriate.

What GAO Found

Several health care and legal factors may make it difficult for consumers to obtain price information for the health care services they receive, particularly estimates of what their complete costs will be. The health care factors include the difficulty of predicting health care services in advance, billing from multiple providers, and the variety of insurance benefit structures. For example, when GAO contacted physicians' offices to obtain information on the price of a diabetes screening, several representatives said the patient needs to be seen by a physician before the physician could determine which screening tests the patient would need. According to provider association officials, consumers may have difficulty obtaining complete cost estimates from providers because providers have to know the status of insured consumers' cost sharing under health benefit plans, such as how much consumers have spent towards their deductible at any given time. In addition to the health care factors, researchers and officials identified several legal factors that may prevent the disclosure of negotiated rates between insurers and providers, which may be used to estimate consumers' complete costs. For example, several insurance company officials GAO interviewed said that contractual obligations with providers may prohibit the sharing of negotiated rates with the insurer's members on their price transparency initiatives' websites. Similarly, some officials and researchers told GAO that providers and insurers may be concerned with sharing negotiated rates due to the proprietary nature of the information and because of antitrust law concerns.

The eight public and private price transparency initiatives GAO examined, selected in part because they provide price information on a specific health care service by provider, vary in the price information they make available to consumers. These initiatives include one administered by HHS, which is also expected to expand its price transparency efforts in the future. The price information made available by the selected initiatives ranges from hospitals' billed charges, which are the amounts hospitals bill for services before any discounts are applied, to prices based on insurance companies' contractually negotiated rates with providers, to prices based on claims data that report payments made to a provider for that service. The price information varies, in large part, due to limits reported by the initiatives in their access or authority to collect certain price data. In addition to price information, most of the selected initiatives also provide a variety of nonprice information, such as quality data on providers, for consumers to consider along with price when making decisions about a provider. Lastly, GAO found that two of the selected initiatives—one publicly available with information only for a particular state and one available to members of a health insurance plan—are able to provide an estimate of a consumer's complete cost. The two initiatives are able to provide this information in part because of the type of data to which they have access—claims data and negotiated rates, respectively. For the remaining initiatives, they either do not use more meaningful price data or are constrained by other factors, including concerns about disclosing what providers may consider proprietary information. As HHS continues and expands its price transparency efforts, it has opportunities to promote more complete cost estimates for consumers.

ABBREVIATIONS

AHRQ	Agency for Healthcare Research and Quality
APCD	All Payer Claims Database
CMS	Centers for Medicare and Medicaid Services
CPT	Current Procedural Terminology
DOJ	Department of Justice
FEHB	Federal Employee Health Benefits
FTC	Federal Trade Commission
HHS	Department of Health and Human Services

OPM	Office of Personnel Management
PPACA	Patient Protection and Affordable Care Act
WHA	Wisconsin Hospital Association

September 23, 2011
Congressional Requesters

Health care spending increased in recent years by an average of nearly 7 percent per year, from $1.4 trillion in 2000 to $2.5 trillion in 2009.[1] Consumers are becoming responsible for a growing proportion of this spending, such as in the case of those with insurance who face increased use of high-deductible health plans and other forms of cost sharing.[2] For example, from 2006 to 2010, the percentage of covered workers enrolled in high-deductible health plans increased from 4 percent to 13 percent, and the percentage of covered workers with a deductible of $1,000 or more for single coverage almost tripled, from 10 percent to 27 percent.[3] Depending upon the insurance plan, insured consumers are generally responsible for the cost of health care services until their deductible has been met. Even after reaching their deductibles, consumers may face significant out-of-pocket costs, such as fees associated with care received from a physician, laboratory, or hospital that are outside of an insurance network and may also bill for their services separately. Consumers without health insurance are also responsible for the cost of their care, and without a third party to negotiate on their behalf these consumers are generally responsible for paying what the provider charges, minus any agreed-to discounts, rather than discounted rates negotiated between the insurer and provider.

Consumers generally learn of their health care costs after receiving care, such as when they receive a bill from their provider or an explanation of benefits from their insurer. In contrast, information on health care prices is considered transparent when this information is available to consumers before they receive health care services.[4] Transparent health care price information may help consumers anticipate their health care costs and reduce the possibility of unexpected expenses. When accompanied by information on the quality of care, transparent price information may also help consumers make more informed choices about their care. Specifically, research suggests that health care price transparency is most relevant for consumers who are having services that can be planned for in advance.[5] Researchers have identified characteristics of the most meaningful types of transparent price information, such as information that includes estimates of what the complete cost will be to a consumer for a service or services.[6] Based on this research, we define an estimate of a consumer's complete health care cost as price information on a health care service or services that (1) reflects any negotiated discounts; (2) is inclusive of all costs to the consumer associated with a service or services, including hospital, physician, and lab fees; and (3) identifies a consumer's out-of-pocket cost.

In recent years various federal, state, and private sector efforts have been initiated to make health care price information available to consumers. Federal efforts include various price transparency initiatives administered by the Department of Health and Human Services (HHS) and Centers for Medicare and Medicaid Services (CMS) that provide price information on health care services, prescription drugs, and health insurance plans. For example, HHS provides price information on insurance plans, such as the amount of cost-sharing and premium rates for specific plans, through its healthcare.gov website. In addition, CMS's Medicare Plan Finder provides information on prescription drug prices, and CMS's Health Care Consumer Initiatives provide information on the price Medicare pays for common health care services by various geographic areas.[7] At the state level, the National Conference of State Legislatures reports that at least 30 states have proposed or enacted some form of price transparency legislation,[8] and a report by America's Health Insurance Plans, an industry group, states that at least 25 states have price transparency initiatives that provide publicly accessible websites with health care price information.[9] Additionally, with the enactment of the Patient Protection and Affordable Care Act (PPACA) in 2010, hospitals operating in the United States are required annually to make public and update a list of their hospital's standard charges for items and services provided by the hospital.[10]

In addition to existing price transparency initiatives, more efforts are planned that may increase the amount of health care price information available to consumers. For example, under PPACA, Health Insurance Exchanges for each state must be developed by January 1, 2014, to facilitate the purchase of qualified health plans and assist small employers in facilitating enrollment of their employees in these health plans.[11] The Exchanges must require participating health plans to permit individuals to learn through a website or other means the amount of cost sharing, such as deductibles and copayments, for which they would be responsible when receiving specific health care services if covered under each company's insurance plan.[12]

In light of consumers' increased responsibility for paying the costs of their health care and efforts aimed at making price information transparent, you asked us to study the extent to which health care price information actually is available to consumers and other interested parties. This report describes (1) how various factors affect the availability of health care price information for consumers and (2) the information selected public and private health care price transparency initiatives make available to consumers and other interested parties.

To describe how various factors affect the availability of health care price information for consumers, we reviewed relevant literature, such as reports from the Congressional Budget Office and the Center for Studying Health System Change.[13] In addition to reviewing relevant literature, we interviewed researchers who have expertise in health care price transparency;[14] a selection of hospital, physician, and insurer associations; officials from two of the largest insurance companies by enrollment; and officials from the selected public and private price transparency initiatives in the authors' review. In their review of relevant literature and interviews with officials, the authors focused on identifying factors that affect the availability of health care price information, including estimates of complete costs to consumers. To provide illustrative examples of how the factors we identified may affect the availability of health care price information, including estimates of consumers' complete costs, and to gain the perspective of consumers on this issue, we anonymously contacted representatives from 39 providers—19 hospitals and 20 primary care physician offices. From these providers we requested price information on two selected health care services: full knee replacement surgery and diabetes screening. We randomly selected these hospitals and physicians from a health care market in Colorado, which requires certain providers to make price information on selected services available to consumers upon request.[15] We did not assess the accuracy of the price information provided by these selected providers, nor did we evaluate the effectiveness of Colorado's law. (See app. I for more information about the authors' methodology for selecting and contacting hospitals and physicians and the information we obtained.)

To describe the information selected public and private price transparency initiatives make available to consumers and other interested parties, we judgmentally selected a total of eight price transparency initiatives that met the authors' definition of a price transparency initiative— initiatives that make provider-specific price information on a specific health care service available to consumers and other interested parties.[16]

Specifically, the authors' eight selected initiatives include: one federal price transparency initiative, which was the only federal price transparency initiative we identified that met the authors' definition;[17] five state initiatives,[18] which we selected based on input from researchers with subject-matter expertise and on the initiatives' geographic variation; and two private initiatives, which we selected from among those provided by the top 10 insurance companies by enrollment in 2009 and based upon input from researchers with subject-matter expertise.[19] See table 1 for a summary of the eight public and private initiatives that we selected.

Table 1. Selected Public and Private Sector Price Transparency Initiatives

Type of initiative	Administrating entity and name of price transparency initiative
Public (federal)	Centers for Medicare and Medicaid Services Hospital Compare
Public (state)	California Common Surgeries and Charges Comparison
	Florida Health Finder
	Massachusetts MyHealthCareOptions
	New Hampshire HealthCost
	Wisconsin Hospital Association PricePointa
Private	Aetna Member Payment Estimator
	Anthem Care Comparison

Source: GAO.

[a]In some cases, a statewide initiative is administered by a private third party entity, such as a state hospital association, but the state has a role in its initiation, regulation, or ongoing development of the price transparency initiative. In these cases, we have classified these as "public (state) initiatives" for the purpose of our review.

For each of the eight initiatives we selected, we interviewed officials and reviewed documentation to identify the types of health care price and other information these initiatives make available—including the extent to which the initiatives make available price information that includes estimates of consumers' complete costs for health care services. As part of this documentation review, we also reviewed the information available to consumers on the selected initiatives' websites.

We conducted this performance audit from November 2010 to September 2011, in accordance with generally accepted government auditing standards. Those standards require that we plan and perform the audit to obtain sufficient, appropriate evidence to provide a reasonable basis for our findings and conclusions based on our audit objectives. We believe that the evidence obtained provides a reasonable basis for our findings and conclusions based on our audit objectives.

BACKGROUND

Research indicates that making price and other contextual information available is important for consumers to be able to anticipate the costs of their care and also to make informed health care decisions. In recent years, many public and private price transparency initiatives have been initiated to provide consumers with information about the price of their health care services.

Health Care Pricing

Determining the price of a health care service often involves coordination between providers, insurers, and consumers. Providers, such as hospitals or physicians, charge consumers fees for the services they receive, which are known as billed charges. Payers, such as insurance companies, often have contractual agreements with providers under which the payers negotiate lower payment rates for a service on behalf of their members or beneficiaries. These rates are known as negotiated rates. In the case of Medicare specifically, CMS sets the program's payment rates for providers based on a formula that includes several factors, such as geographic location.

For consumers with health insurance, their out-of-pocket costs for a health care service is determined by the amount of cost sharing specified in the benefits of their health insurance plan for services covered by the insurer. For consumers who lack health insurance, they are often billed for the full amount charged by the provider, such as a billed charge from a hospital. The estimated out-of-pocket cost for an uninsured consumer will typically be the billed charge for a health care service minus any charity care or discounts that may be applied by the provider.[20]

Health Care Services and Episodes of Care

Providers and payers often price health care services using the various codes used by health care professionals. For example, physicians may bill for their services based on Current Procedural Terminology (CPT) codes developed by the American Medical Association. Individual health care services, such as those referred to by individual CPT codes, can be grouped or bundled together into an episode of care, which refers to a group of health care services associated with a patient's condition over a defined period of time. An episode of care for a knee replacement, for example, includes multiple services such as those provided during the actual surgery, as well as preoperation and postoperation consultations.

The episode of care would also include services provided by various providers who typically bill separately, such as a hospital, surgeon, and anesthesiologist. PPACA requires HHS to develop a national pilot program, which may include bundled payments for episodes of care surrounding certain hospitalizations, in order to improve the coordination, quality, and efficiency of health care services.[21]

Importance of Quality and Other Contextual Information

According to researchers, it is important for consumers to have access to quality of care and other information to provide context to the price information and help consumers in their decision making. For example, according to the Agency for Healthcare Research and Quality (AHRQ),[22] appropriate quality of care information for consumers may include the mortality rates for a specific procedure, the percentage of patients with surgical complications or postoperative infections, or the average length of stay, among other measures.[23] By combining quality and price information, some researchers argue that consumers can then use this information to choose providers with the highest quality and the lowest price—thereby obtaining the greatest value when purchasing care.[24] Furthermore, some research suggests that information on volume (the number of services performed) may be used as an indication of quality for certain procedures.[25] This assumes a positive association between the number of times a provider administers a service and the quality of the service provided. Information about previous patients' satisfaction with a provider's service can also help consumers make decisions about their health care.

Development and Use of Public and Private Price Transparency Initiatives

Public price transparency initiatives often began in response to laws or orders requiring an agency or organization to make price information available to consumers, while private sector initiatives started primarily through voluntary efforts. For example, in response to a 2006 federal executive order to promote quality and efficiency in federal health care programs, federal agencies that administer or sponsor a health care program were directed, among other things, to make available to enrollees the prices paid for health care services.[26] In response, agencies including HHS (including its component agencies such as CMS and AHRQ) and OPM began to make health care price information available. Similarly, over 30 states have proposed or enacted some type of price transparency legislation, though what is actually required varies greatly across the states.[27] For example, some states, such as Colorado and South Dakota, require hospitals to disclose, upon request, the expected or average price for the treatment requested.[28] In contrast, some states, such as Maine and Minnesota, require that certain health care price information be made publicly available through an Internet website.[29] While many public price transparency initiatives began as a result of legislation, private sector price transparency initiatives, such as insurance company initiatives, were established voluntarily for various reasons. For example, insurance officials that we spoke with said their price transparency initiatives started for reasons such as increased interest from employers to curb costs, to gain a competitive edge over other insurance companies without price transparency initiatives, and to help their members become better health care consumers. Other private price transparency initiatives, such as Health Care Blue Book and PriceDoc, were started to help consumers find and negotiate fair prices for health care services.[30]

Though both public and private price transparency initiatives have become more widespread in the last 5 years, some research suggests that even if consumers have access to price information, such as price information made available by these initiatives, they may not use such information in their decision making.[31] For example, insured consumers may be less sensitive to prices, since the financial costs of selecting one provider over another may be borne by the insurer, not the consumer. Despite these concerns, some research indicates that consumers want access to price information before they receive health care services and have tried to use price information to some degree to inform their decision making.[32] Furthermore, research states that incentives may be helpful to further consumers' use of transparent price information. Specifically, financial incentives may include insurers providing lower out-of-pocket costs for their members if they select low-price, high-quality providers.[33]

VARIOUS HEALTH CARE AND LEGAL FACTORS MAKE ESTIMATES OF CONSUMERS' COMPLETE COSTS DIFFICULT TO OBTAIN

Several health care and legal factors can make it difficult for consumers to obtain price information—in particular, estimates of their complete costs—for health care services before the services are provided. The health care factors include the difficulty of predicting in advance all the services that will be provided for an episode of care and billing services from multiple providers separately. In addition, according to researchers and officials we interviewed, legal factors, such as contractual obligations, may prevent insurers and providers from making available their negotiated rates, which can be used to estimate consumers' complete costs.

Various Factors, Such as the Difficulty of Predicting Health Care Services in Advance, Billing from Multiple Providers, and the Variety of Insurance Benefit Structures, Can Make Estimates of Consumers' Complete Costs Difficult to Obtain

One factor that may make it difficult for consumers to obtain estimates of their complete costs for a health care service is that it may be difficult for providers to predict which services a patient will need in advance. Specifically, physicians often do not decide what services their patients will need until after examining them. Researchers and officials we spoke with commented that health care services are not standardized across all patients because of each patient's unique circumstances, which influence the specific services a physician would recommend. For example, when we anonymously contacted 20 physicians' offices to obtain information on the price of a diabetes screening, several representatives said the patient needs to be seen by a physician before the physician would know what tests the patient would need.[34]

In addition, even after identifying what health care service or services a patient may need, additional aspects associated with the delivery of a service may be difficult to predict in advance, such as the length of time a patient stays in a hospital. This factor can make it challenging for providers to estimate consumers' complete costs in advance. For example, when we anonymously contacted 19 hospitals to obtain information on the price of a full knee replacement surgery, several hospital representatives quoted a range of prices, from about $33,000 to about $101,000. The representatives explained that the price for the procedure could vary based on a variety of factors, such as the time the patient will be in the operating room and the type of anesthetic the patient may receive, and some noted that they would need to know this information if they were to provide a more specific price estimate.

Several hospital and physician office representatives we spoke with recommended that insured consumers contact their insurer for complete cost information; however, the inability to predict which health care services will be needed in advance also makes it challenging for insurers to provide complete cost estimates. Officials from an insurer association commented that, if asked by their members for cost estimates, insurance company representatives may require more information—such as the CPT codes for the services a patient will receive—before the insurers can provide a cost estimate. However, in the instances when providers cannot predict in advance the codes for which they will bill, consumers will be unable to provide the respective codes to insurers and obtain complete cost estimates from them.

Another factor is that many services included in one episode of care may be provided by multiple providers, such as a hospital and surgeon, who bill for their services separately. This makes obtaining complete cost information challenging because, in these cases, consumers may have to contact multiple providers to obtain estimates of their complete costs. Many providers can only give price estimates in advance for the services that they provide, and are often unaware of the prices for services performed by other providers. For example, when we contacted hospitals anonymously for the price of a full knee replacement, none were able to provide information on the complete cost to consumers for this service. The hospital representatives we contacted who could provide price information were only able to provide us with the hospital's estimated charges or a Medicare deductible amount for the service and could not provide us with the charges associated with the other providers involved in the service, such as a surgeon or anesthesiologist. Charges from these providers are typically billed separately from the hospital's charges, even though some of these services are provided in the hospital. Similarly, when we called physicians' offices to obtain information on the price of a diabetes screening, most representatives could not tell us how much the associated lab fees would cost and some noted that this was because the lab fees are billed separately. Several hospital and physician office representatives we spoke with suggested we contact the other providers, such as a surgeon or lab, separately in order to obtain information on the price of these services. However, officials from a provider association questioned how consumers would even know which providers to contact to get price information if the consumers do not know all of the different providers who are involved in an episode of care in advance. Lastly, consumers may have difficulty obtaining complete cost estimates from providers because providers are often unaware of these costs due to the variety of insured consumers' health benefit structures. For example, according to officials from a provider association, physicians may have difficulty accessing insured consumers' health benefit plan information, and thus may not be able to provide estimates of consumers' out-of-pocket costs under their specific benefit plans. For example, officials stated that for physicians to inform a patient about the price of a health care service in advance they have to know the status of consumers' cost sharing under their specific health benefit plan, such as how much consumers have spent in out-of-pocket costs or towards their deductible at any given time. Without this information, physicians may have difficulty providing accurate out-of-pocket estimates for insured consumers. In addition, different consumers may have out-of-pocket costs that vary within the same benefit plan, which adds to the variety of potential costs a patient could have, and creates complexity for providers in providing complete cost estimates to consumers. Officials from provider associations commented that insurers should be responsible for providing complete cost information to their insured customers because insurers can provide price information specific to insured consumers' situations. However, insurers may also have difficulty estimating consumers' complete costs. Specifically, according to a 2007 report by the Healthcare Financial Management Association, many insurers do not have data systems that are capable of calculating real-time estimates of complete costs for their members prior to receiving a service.[35] As a result, insurers may have difficulty maintaining real-time data on how much their members have paid towards their deductibles, which could affect an estimate of the complete cost.

Additionally, according to officials from an insurance company, it is difficult for insurers to estimate complete costs when insured customers receive services from providers that are outside of the insurer's network. These estimates may be difficult to provide because insurers have not negotiated a rate with providers out of the insurer's network, and thus may be unaware of these providers' billed charges before a service is given. Officials from an insurance company explained that this concern is especially a problem for their members who go to an in-network hospital and are seen by a nonparticipating physician within that hospital during their visit. The officials explained that this can occur without the patient's knowledge because patients often do not choose certain providers, such as radiologists or anesthesiologists, and consumers may be faced with significant out-of-pocket costs.

Researchers and Officials Identify Legal Factors That May Prevent the Disclosure of Negotiated Rates, Which Can Be Used to Estimate Consumers' Complete Costs

Researchers and officials we interviewed identified several legal factors that may prevent providers and insurers from sharing negotiated rates, which can be used to estimate consumers' complete costs. First, some officials stated that some contractual obligations between insurers and providers prohibit the disclosure of negotiated rates with anyone outside of the contracting entities, such as an insurer's members.[36] Specifically, most officials representing insurance companies have reported that some hospitals have included contractual obligations in their agreements with insurers that restrict insurers from disclosing negotiated rates to their members. For example, some insurance company officials we interviewed told us that these contractual obligations prohibited the sharing of specific information on negotiated rates between providers and insurers on their price transparency initiatives' websites. Officials from one insurance company said that they generally accept these contractual obligations, particularly in the case of hospitals that have significant market leverage, because they do not want to exclude these hospitals from their networks.[37] Second, some of the officials and researchers we spoke with reported that providers and insurers may be concerned with sharing their negotiated rates, considered proprietary information, which may be protected by law from unauthorized disclosure. Some officials and researchers we spoke with suggest that without these rates, it could be more difficult for consumers to obtain complete cost estimates. According to officials from an insurer association, proprietary information such as negotiated rates may be prohibited from being shared under the Uniform Trade Secrets Act, which many states have adopted to protect the competitive advantage of the entities involved.[38] These laws are designed to protect against the wrongful disclosure or wrongful appropriation of trade secrets, which may include negotiated rates. For example, if a hospital was aware that another hospital negotiated a higher rate with the same insurance company, then the lower-priced hospital could seek out higher negotiated rates which may eliminate the first hospital's competitive advantage. Conversely, if officials from an insurance company were aware that another insurer paid the same hospital a lower rate for a given service, the higher-paying insurer may try to negotiate lower payment rates with that hospital. Lastly, some researchers and officials noted that antitrust law concerns may discourage providers and insurers from making negotiated rates public.[39] For example, some insurance company officials we spoke with expressed concerns that sharing negotiated rates publicly would give multiple competing providers access to each other's rates, and therefore could lead to collusion in price negotiations between providers and insurers.[40] According to the Federal Trade Commission (FTC) and the Department of Justice (DOJ)—the principal federal agencies enforcing the antitrust laws—antitrust laws aim to protect and promote competition by preventing businesses from acting together in ways that can limit competition. Joint guidance from FTC and DOJ indicates that without appropriate safeguards, exchanges of price information—which insurance company officials told us could include negotiated rates—among competing providers may present the risk that competing providers communicate with each other regarding a mutually acceptable level of prices for health care services or compensation for employees.[41] Although some officials and researchers noted that antitrust laws may discourage making negotiated rates public, the FTC and DOJ guidance also identifies circumstances in which exchanges of health care price information—that could include negotiated rates—are unlikely to raise significant antitrust concerns. These circumstances require the collecting of price information by a third-party entity and ensuring that any information disseminated is aggregated such that it would not allow recipients to identify the prices charged by an individual provider.[42] Under these circumstances, consumers may not be hindered in their ability to have information that will allow them to make informed decisions about their health care.

SELECTED INITIATIVES VARY IN THE INFORMATION THEY MAKE AVAILABLE, AND FEW INITIATIVES PROVIDE ESTIMATES OF CONSUMERS' COMPLETE COSTS

The price information made available to consumers by the eight selected price transparency initiatives varies, in large part due to differences in the price data available to each initiative. Additionally, we found that few of the selected initiatives are able to provide estimates of consumers' complete costs, primarily due to limitations of the price data that they use and other obstacles.

Selected Initiatives Vary in the Information They Make Available to Consumers and Other Interested Parties

The eight public and private price transparency initiatives that we examined vary in the price information they make available to consumers. (See table 2.) Three public initiatives in California, Florida, and Wisconsin make information available on hospitals' billed charges, which are typically the amounts hospitals bill payers and patients for services before any negotiated or reduced payment discounts are applied. In general, hospitals' billed charges do not reflect the amount most payers and patients ultimately pay for the service. Two private initiatives administered by Aetna and Anthem provide their members with price information based on their contracts with providers, and this information reflects the insurer's negotiated discounts. Similarly, the federal initiative provides price information based on Medicare payment rates. Initiatives in Massachusetts and New Hampshire provide price information, based on payments made to providers, using claims data, and these prices reflect any negotiated discounts or other reductions off the billed charges.[43] Despite differences in the types of price information they provide, the selected initiatives are generally similar in the types of services for which they provided price information,[44] with most providing price information only for a limited set of hospital or surgical services that are common, comparable, or planned in advance, such as a knee replacement or a diagnostic test.[45]

Various factors help explain the differences in the types of price information made available by the selected initiatives. In some cases, the initiatives provide certain types of price information because of the price data available to them, generally through state law. For example, the Wisconsin initiative provides price information based on hospitals' billed charges because the state contracted with the Wisconsin Hospital Association (WHA) to collect and disseminate hospital information, including hospitals' billed charges, when the state privatized hospital data collection. WHA saw this as an opportunity to develop a price transparency initiative that reported billed charges for consumers.[46] In both California and Florida, initiative officials said that state laws enabled the state to collect and make hospitals' billed charges public and this gave the states the authority to make this information available to consumers.[47] In Massachusetts, officials said that 2006 state health reform legislation provided the state with the necessary authority to collect claims data for the price transparency initiative.[48]

Table 2. Types of Health Care Services and Price Information Made Available by Selected Price Transparency Initiatives, 2011

Selected price transparency initiatives	Health care services for which price information is made available[a]	Type of price information made available
Centers for Medicare and Medicaid Services (CMS) Hospital Compare	43 common inpatient hospital services	Median Medicare payment rates[b]
California Common Surgeries and Charges Comparison	37 inpatient surgical services	Median billed charges from hospitalsc
Florida Health Finder	Over 150 inpatient, outpatient, and ambulatory surgery center services	Range (25th to 75th percentile) of billed charges from hospitals[c]
Massachusetts MyHealthCareOptions	37 inpatient and outpatient hospital services	Median and range (15th to 85th percentile) of insurers' aggregated payments made to that provider based on claims data[d]
New Hampshire HealthCost	42 preventative health, emergency visits, radiology, surgical procedures, and maternity services	Median payment made by that specific insurance plan to that specific provider based on claims data[d]
Wisconsin Hospital Association PricePoint	316 inpatient hospital services, 75 outpatient surgical services, and 27 emergency department and urgent care services	Average and median billed charges from hospitals and median and range (20th to 80th percentile) of billed charges from ambulatory care centers[c]
Aetna Member Payment Estimator	40 hospital service bundles and 460 physician service bundles (comprised of 3 categories of physician office visits, surgical procedures, and diagnostic tests and procedures)	Aetna's negotiated rates[e]
Anthem Care Comparison	59 service bundles including hospital inpatient and outpatient services, physician office visits, and diagnostic and imaging services	Range of Anthem's negotiated rates[e]

Source: GAO analysis of selected price transparency initiatives and interviews with administering officials.

[a]The selected price transparency initiatives use different terms to refer to what we describe as the health care "services" for which consumers can look up price information.

[b]Medicare payment rates are the prices CMS recently paid providers for services provided to Medicare beneficiaries. These payment rates are set by CMS and based on various factors such as geographic location.

[c]Billed charges are the amount hospitals and other providers bill payers and patients for a service, before any negotiated or reduced payment discounts are applied, and thus generally do not reflect the amount most payers and patients ultimately pay for the service.

[d]Claims data reflect the amount, based on the record of payments made by consumers and payers, a provider was previously reimbursed for the service and incorporates any insurer's negotiated discounts or any reduced discounts given. Initiatives used claims data to identify and report price information in different ways. New Hampshire's price transparency website uses its claims data to report a single point estimate of the estimated cost of the service, based on the median of all payments paid by that specific insurance plan to that provider for that service. Massachusetts's price transparency website combines the claims of all the applicable insurers and reports a price reflecting the aggregated price per provider for that service, as paid by these insurers.

[e]Negotiated rates are the prices an insurance company has negotiated with a provider to provide a health care service. These prices reflect prices under contract and any discounts that have been agreed to.

In other cases, the price information the initiatives provide reflects choices made by initiative officials regarding the types of information that they considered would be most helpful to consumers. For example, in developing Hospital Compare, CMS officials chose to provide price information based on Medicare payment rates to hospitals because, according to officials, this information would be more helpful than hospitals' retrospective billed charges for Medicare patients. The officials explained that hospitals' billed charges are too divergent from what Medicare and insurance companies actually pay for the same service, and CMS officials reasoned that Medicare rates could give consumers, particularly those without insurance, a point of comparison from which they may be able to negotiate lower prices with providers.[49] In New Hampshire, officials said they successfully sought legislation to get access to claims data from all payers in the state to establish an All Payer Claims Database (APCD) for their initiative.[50] Based on an earlier experience with posting billed charges and feedback from consumers, New Hampshire officials were convinced that billed charges were not useful for insured consumers.

Additionally, some factors that may limit access to certain price data also limit how the price information is presented to consumers. For example, some of the selected initiatives, such as Florida and Anthem, present price information as a range, which avoids providing a specific price that providers may consider proprietary.[51] Anthem officials further noted that the primary reason the initiative provides price information as a range is so that the price information can better reflect for consumers the billing variation and differences in treatment decisions that occur when health care services are delivered to different patients. In Massachusetts, the initiative combines the claims, or prices paid, by commercial insurers for that specific hospital service and reports a provider's median price as well as a range of prices paid for that service. Officials explained that they present aggregated price information across all health plans to avoid disclosing prices that may raise proprietary concerns among providers and insurers. In another approach, the two initiatives by New Hampshire and Aetna bundle multiple services typically performed at the same time into the price presented, such as bundling all associated costs for a hip replacement surgery. By doing so, New Hampshire officials said that they are able to mask the specific rates paid for individual items, and avoid proprietary concerns, while providing an easily understandable estimate for the total health care service. Lastly, officials from the Aetna and Anthem initiatives cited provider resistance as limiting the extent to which they can make price information available to their members for all providers in the insurers' networks—with provider-imposed contractual obligations requiring the Aetna and Anthem initiatives to omit price information for certain providers in the initiatives' websites' search results.

In addition to providing the price of a service, most selected initiatives also provide a wide range of nonprice information, such as information on quality of care measures or patient volume. Five of the eight selected initiatives provide quality information for consumers to consider along with price when making decisions about a provider. (See table 3.) In addition to providing quality and volume measures, initiatives also shared information, such as resources for understanding and using price information, including explanations of the source and limitations of the price data, glossaries, and medical encyclopedias. Initiatives also provided a range of supplementary financial information to give context to the price information provided. For example, Massachusetts' initiative presents symbols ($, $$, $$$) to indicate how the provider's price compares to the state median for that service in an effort to provide what officials described as more easily understood price information for consumers who are familiar with graphical ratings systems. Additionally, Wisconsin's initiative provides pie charts representing the percentage different payer types—such as private insurers, Medicare, and Medicaid—paid to a specific hospital in relation to the total billed charges, which indicates at an aggregate level the extent of discounts given by payer category.

Table 3. Quality and Volume Information Provided by Selected Price Transparency Initiatives

Selected price transparency initiative	Quality data	Volume data	Examples of quality and volume data[a]
Centers for Medicare and Medicaid Services (CMS) Hospital Compare	I	I	Process of care measures, how many Medicare patients were treated for a service at a given facility
California Common Surgeries and Charges Comparison		I	The number of discharges for a service in a given year
Florida Health Finder	I	I	Patient safety indicators, total number of hospitalizations by service at a facility
Massachusetts MyHealthCareOptions	I	I	Information on patient safety practices, number of patients treated
New Hampshire HealthCost			None
Wisconsin Hospital Association PricePoint		I	The number of discharges for a service in a given year
Aetna Member Payment Estimator	I		Designation of quality and efficiency for hospitals and selected specialists
Anthem Care Comparison	I	I	Mortality rates, number of patients who received that treatment

Source: GAO analysis of selected price transparency initiatives and interviews with administering officials.

[a]Quality data and other nonprice information provided by the initiatives' websites came from a variety of national sources, including WebMD, CMS, Leapfrog Group, and AHRQ. Many state initiatives also relied on information reported to state agencies, such as the California Office of Statewide Health Planning and Development, the Florida Center for Health Information and Policy Analysis, and the Massachusetts Division of Health Care Finance and Policy.

Some officials expressed reservations about how consumers may use price and quality information together.[52] Insurance company officials we spoke with see linking price to quality information as a means for consumers to identify high-value providers and for the company to create more cost-efficient provider networks. In Hospital Compare, however, quality data and price data are not linked. CMS officials said that while quality data are featured prominently on Hospital Compare, price information is featured less prominently. CMS officials explained that promoting price information to consumers, in the absence of greater consumer education about how to understand price information in relation to quality, could lead consumers to select high-priced providers due to an assumption that price is indicative of quality. Due to similar concerns that consumers may assume that a higher price is a sign of higher quality, Aetna's initiative provides information to educate consumers that high quality and low price are not mutually exclusive.

Lastly, in addition to the variety of price and other information made available by the selected initiatives, the initiatives also vary in terms of who has access to the initiatives' websites and in terms of their expected audiences. For example, the price information provided by the federal initiative we selected is available to all consumers through a publicly available website. CMS officials said the expected audience of this initiative includes insured and uninsured consumers, researchers, Medicare beneficiaries, and providers. Like the federal initiative, all of the selected state initiatives' websites are publicly available, although they include price information only for their particular state. In contrast, the price information provided by the two selected insurance company initiatives' websites are accessible to their members, but not to the general public.

Few Selected Initiatives Provide Estimates of Complete Costs to Consumers

Few of the selected initiatives provide estimates of consumers' complete costs, which is price information that incorporates any negotiated discounts; is inclusive of all costs associated with a particular health care service, such as hospital, physician, and lab fees; and identifies consumers' out-of-pocket costs. (See table 4.) Specifically, of our eight selected initiatives, only the Aetna and New Hampshire initiatives provide estimates of a consumer's complete cost. The two initiatives are able to provide this information in part because they have access to and use price data—negotiated rates and claims data, respectively—that allow them to provide consumers with a price for the service by each provider that is inclusive of any negotiated discounts or reduced payments made to the billed charge. Specifically, Aetna bases its price data on its contractual rates with providers, which include negotiated discounts.

Table 4. Extent to Which Selected Price Transparency Initiatives Provide Price Information That Reflects Estimates of Consumers' Complete Costs

	Components of complete cost estimates provided by initiative			
	Price reflects negotiated discounts	**Price inclusive of all associated costs, including hospital, physician, and lab fees**	**Identifies outof-pocket costs**	**Complete cost estimate provided by initiative**
Selected price transparency initiative				
Centers for Medicare and Medicaid Services Hospital Compare	√			
California Common Surgeries and Charges Comparison			a	
Florida Health Finder				
Massachusetts MyHealthCareOptions	√b			
New Hampshire HealthCost	√	√	√c	√
Wisconsin Hospital Association PricePoint			a	
Aetna Member Payment Estimator	√	√	√d	√
Anthem Care Comparison	√	√		

Source: GAO analysis of selected price transparency initiatives' documentation and interviews with administering officials.

[a] Selected initiatives in Florida, Wisconsin, and California report price information as billed charges, that is, the price billed to consumers with no negotiated discounts from insurers or providers included. An uninsured patient may expect to be billed the full amount charged by the provider; however, some research indicates that uninsured patients rarely pay the full billed charge. In practice, what an uninsured consumer may be expected to pay out-of-pocket is often arranged on a case-by-case basis with the provider, and may depend on various factors, such as the consumer's ability to pay, the availability of charity care or sliding scale deductions, and state restrictions on what hospitals can collect from uninsured patients.

[b] Massachusetts's initiative uses the claims data of applicable insurers that reflect payments made after negotiated discounts have been applied. The price presented

is an aggregate of all the prices paid by these insurers to that provider for that service.

[c] For insured consumers, New Hampshire's initiative identifies an estimated out-of-pocket cost, by health plan, for that provider and that service. For uninsured consumers, the New Hampshire initiative reports price information based on billed charges minus a 15 percent discount for uninsured consumers, which it states is a typical uninsured discount.

[d] Aetna's initiative provides out-of-pocket costs only to its intended audience, Aetna members.

New Hampshire provides price information based on its records of closed claims of particular providers for particular services under a consumer's specific health insurance plan.[53] Both initiatives use claims data to identify all of the hospital, physician, and lab fees associated with the services for which they provide price information. For calculating estimated out-of-pocket costs, Aetna links member data to its price transparency website, which automatically updates and calculates the member's estimated out-of-pocket costs in real-time based on the provider and service reported, and the member's partially exhausted deductibles. In contrast, to calculate out-of-pocket costs, insured users of New Hampshire's initiative's website enter their insurance plan, their deductible amount, and their percentage rate of co-insurance. New Hampshire's Health Cost website then uses that information to calculate an out-of-pocket cost, along with a total cost for the service by provider. Both initiatives demonstrate that while providing complete cost information presents challenges, it can be done—either as undertaken by Aetna for its members or as carried out by New Hampshire, which makes complete cost information available through publicly accessible means.

As table 4 shows, six of the eight initiatives that we reviewed do not provide estimates of consumers' complete costs. The reasons for this vary by initiative, but are primarily due to the limitations of the price data that each initiative uses. For example, initiatives in California, Florida, and Wisconsin provide price information based on billed charges from hospitals, which do not reflect discounts negotiated by payers and providers, all associated costs (such as physician fees), and out-of-pocket costs. An official representing Wisconsin's initiative said that WHA commonly receives requests from consumers to include physician fees in the price estimate, but the initiative does not have access to these price data, as they are part of a separate billing process and the hospitals do not have these data to submit. California officials said that collecting claims data from insurers would require additional legal authority, raise proprietary concerns, and pose resource challenges. Florida officials acknowledged that providing a billed charge is not as meaningful for consumers as other types of price data, such as claims data. However, while Florida officials have the authority to collect claims data,[54] they said that at this time they are limited from pursuing such information due to the expected financial costs of collecting and storing the data and the challenges of overcoming the proprietary concerns of providers and insurers. Florida officials characterized their initiative's inability to report out-of-pocket costs as a major limitation. The federal initiative provides price information that reflects what Medicare pays to hospitals for a given service but does not reflect what consumers, including Medicare beneficiaries, would pay out-of-pocket. CMS officials said that providing out-of-pocket costs was too complicated to calculate in advance due to consumers' medical variation and technological limitations.

In contrast, other initiatives have access to data that may enable the initiatives to provide more complete cost estimates to consumers, but certain factors limit the extent to which this type of information is made available. For example, the Massachusetts initiative has access to claims data that could be used to provide more complete cost estimates to consumers, such as negotiated discounts for commercial insurers.[55] However, it presents price information that aggregates the prices paid by commercial insurers for particular services, in part due to insurers' and providers' concerns about the initiative disclosing price information by insurer. As a result, consumers are unable to see an estimate for a particular provider that is specific to their insurance company or to calculate their out-of pocket costs based on their specific plan. The officials noted that providers' and insurers' resistance to publicly reporting payments made by insurers may also be a challenge for states seeking access to more meaningful price information for their initiatives, such as claims data. Lastly, Anthem's initiative does provide a price inclusive of all associated fees and negotiated discounts, but currently does not use the specific details of consumers' insurance plan benefits, such as their deductible, copayment, or coinsurance, to estimate consumers' out-of-pocket costs.[56]

Conclusion

Transparent health care price information—especially estimates of consumers' complete costs—can be difficult for consumers to obtain prior to receiving care. For example, when we contacted hospitals and physicians to obtain price information for two common services, we generally received only incomplete estimates, which are insufficient for helping consumers to anticipate all of the costs associated with these services or to make more informed decisions about their health care. Our review identified various health care and legal factors that can make it difficult for consumers to obtain meaningful health care price information, such as estimates of consumers' complete costs, in advance of receiving services. This lack of health care price transparency presents a serious challenge for consumers who are increasingly being asked to pay a greater share of their health care costs.

Despite the complexities of doing so, two of the eight price transparency initiatives we examined were able to make complete cost estimates available to consumers. Making meaningful health care price information available to consumers is important, and the fact that two initiatives have been able to do it suggests that this is an attainable goal. To promote health care price transparency, HHS is currently supporting various efforts to make price information available to consumers—including the CMS initiative in our review—and the agency is expected to do more in this area in the future. We note in our review, for example, that HHS provides price information on insurance plans through its healthcare.gov website. Similarly, CMS's web-based Medicare Part D Plan Finder also provides information on prescription drug prices and CMS's Health Care Consumer Initiatives provide information on the price Medicare pays for common health care services at the county and state levels. In the near future, HHS's price transparency efforts are expected to expand. For example, PPACA requires HHS to provide oversight and guidance for the Exchanges that are expected to provide certain price information for consumers through participating insurers. PPACA also directs HHS to develop a pilot program which may include bundled payments, providing another possible opportunity for price transparency. In total, HHS has several opportunities to promote greater health care price transparency for consumers.

Recommendations for Executive Action

As HHS implements its current and forthcoming efforts to make transparent price information available to consumers, we recommend that HHS take the following two actions:

- Determine the feasibility of making estimates of complete costs of health care services available to consumers through any of these efforts.
- Determine, as appropriate, the next steps for making estimates of complete costs of health care services available to consumers.

AGENCY COMMENTS

HHS reviewed a draft of this report and provided technical comments, which we incorporated as appropriate.

Linda T. Kohn
Director, Health Care

APPENDIX I: METHODOLOGY AND RESULTS OF CONTACTING SELECTED PROVIDERS FOR PRICE INFORMATION

To obtain illustrative examples of factors that influence the availability of health care price information for consumers, we anonymously contacted hospitals and primary care physicians with zip codes located in the Denver, Colorado, health care market.[1] We requested the price of a full knee replacement from hospitals and the price of a diabetes screening from primary care physicians. We requested these prices for patients without insurance and for patients with Medicare (without supplemental health insurance). Specifically, we called 19 hospitals and 20 primary care physicians between February 28 and March 10, 2011, and contacted each provider up to three times in an attempt to get a response.[2] We determined that we obtained a response from representatives if they answered the phone or they transferred us to a price quote voice mail message that requested specific information from us about the requested service so representatives could call back with cost estimates. In cases where we were asked to provide more information, such as in the case of receiving a price quote voice mail, we did not provide such information in order to help maintain our anonymity. We considered hospitals and physicians nonresponsive if no one answered the phone, or if we received a voice mail message that did not indicate what we needed to provide in order to receive price information, in all three attempts.

Results from Contacting Hospital Representatives

We received a response from representatives at 17 of the 19 hospitals we contacted. Of the 17 hospital representatives that responded, 10 did not provide any type of price information. None of the hospital representatives could provide a complete cost estimate for a full knee replacement, meaning the price given was not reflective of any negotiated discounts, was not inclusive of all associated costs, and did not identify consumers' out-of-pocket costs. Almost all of the hospital representatives that responded (14 of 17) required more information from us to provide a complete cost estimate, such as current procedural terminology (CPT)[3] codes, the length of time in the operating room, the model of knee used, or what kind of anesthetic would be provided, which we did not provide. Of the 7 hospital representatives that were able to provide some price information, 5 provided billed charges in either a range, such as between $32,974.73 and $100,676.50 or an average charge, such as $82,390, which is typically reflective of what an uninsured consumer would pay.[4] (See table 5 for more information.)

Results from Contacting Physician Office Representatives

We received a response from 18 of the 20 representatives we contacted. Of the physician representatives that responded, most could provide some type of price information (14 of 18), but only 4 out of 18 representatives who responded could provide a complete cost estimate for a diabetes screening. Most representatives who responded (13 of 18) required more information from us to provide a complete cost estimate, such as a diagnosis from a physician and the amount the laboratory would charge, which we did not provide. Additionally, almost half (8 of 18) of representatives who responded said the patient needs to be seen by a physician before determining a complete cost estimate. All 14 physician representatives who were able to provide some type of price information provided price information based on billed charges.[5] (See table 6 for more information.)

Table 5. Results of Contacting Hospitals for the Price of a Full Knee Replacement on Behalf of a Patient with Medicare and without Health Insurance from Those Who Responded

Hospital number and insurance status		Type of priceprovided	Actual price provided	Price reflective of consumers' complete costestimates (Y/N)?	Examples of responses from representativesa
1.	Medicare	Deductible	$1,132 (inpatient services) and $162 (outpatient services) and 20% of Medicare approved amount	N – Does not include associated fees	Representative did not know what the surgeon would charge.
2.	Medicare	Average and range of billed charges, Medicare-allowable amount	$82,390 or $65,000 - $95,000; with Medicare: $13,360 to 16,650.	N – Does not include associated fees or identify out-of-pocket costs	The charges vary depending upon length of stay (2-4 days), length of time in operating room, and model of knee used.
3.	Medicare	None	N/A	N/A	It would take a week to get an estimate after speaking with a nurse.
4.	Medicare	None	N/A	N/A	Asked to leave message with name, date of procedure, physician's name, procedure, and phone number and they will call back with an estimate.
5.	Medicare	None	N/A	N/A	Asked to leave message with name, phone number, CPT codes, physician's name, insurance company name, subscriber's identification number, and date of birth.

Hospital number and insurance status		Type of priceprovided	Actual price provided	Price reflective of consumers' complete costestimates (Y/N)?	Examples of responses from representativesa
6.	Medicare	None	N/A	N/A	Requested us to ask the physician for CPT codes, and provide physician's name. The estimate would only include the hospital facility fees, and unsure what the other charges would be.
7.	Medicare	Deductible	$1,132	N – Does not reflect negotiated rates or include associated fees	Could not provide a charge for the procedure. The deductible does not include physician, rehabilitation, or anesthesiology fees.
8.	Medicare	None	N/A	N/A	Requested CPT codes, how long the length of stay would be in the hospital, how long the patient would be in the operating room, and under what kind of anesthetic (local or general).
9.	Medicare	Range of billed charges, co-payment, and deductible	$32,974.73 to $100,676.50; with Medicare: $2,662 to $2,566 and $1,100 deductible	N – Does not include associated fees	Hospital charges vary based on how many days patient is in the hospital and variation in cases. Representative provided a disclaimer that the price is just an estimate and the hospital is not liable for any differences.
10.	Medicare	Average billed charge and deductible	$50,000 and $1,132	N – Does not reflect negotiated rates and does not include associated fees	Did not provide.

Table 5. (Continued)

Hospital number and insurance status		Type of priceprovided	Actual price provided	Price reflective of consumers' complete costestimates (Y/N)?	Examples of responses from representativesa
11.	Uninsured	None	N/A	N/A	Asked to leave message with name, phone number, procedure, CPT and International Statistical Classification of Diseases (ICD)-9 codes, and date of service. The representative said no one else could provide this information because it is complicated and they would need to check information with the patient's insurer.
12.	Uninsured	None	N/A	N/A	Needed the procedure and diagnostic codes, the name of the hospital, name, phone number, and insurance information.
13.	Uninsured	None	N/A	N/A	Asked to leave message with first and last name, phone number, CPT code (can get from physician), physician's name, insurance company name, subscriber's identification number, and date of birth.
14.	Uninsured	Range of billed charges	$65,000 to $95,000	N – Does not include associated feesb	Range of billed charges is dependent on the model of implant used, number of days in hospital, and how long the operating room time is.

Hospital number and insurance status		Type of priceprovided	Actual price provided	Price reflective of consumers' complete costestimates (Y/N)?	Examples of responses from representativesa
15.	Uninsured	Average billed charge	$58,581.59 (including a discount for self-payers) or $50,023.42 if paid within 4 days of receiving the bill	N – Does not include associated fees	Did not provide.
16.	Uninsured	None	N/A	N/A	Asked to leave message with phone number, patient name, procedure, CPT code, ICD-9 code, and date of service (if scheduled).
17.	Uninsured	None	N/A	N/A	Recommended we contact an orthopedic surgeon or physician for price information.

Source: GAO analysis of anonymous phone calls to hospitals.

[a]When we called several hospitals we received a price quote voice mail message which asked us to list information, such as diagnosis codes for the service we inquired about and personal information, and a representative would call back with a cost estimate. We considered this receiving a response since this method was the way these hospitals responded to such requests. In cases where we were asked to provide additional information by a voice mail or representative, we did not provide such information in order to help maintain our anonymity.

[b]According to the hospital representative we spoke with, the range of billed charges provided were considered an out-of-pocket cost for an uninsured consumer.

Table 6. Results of Contacting Physicians for the Price of a Diabetes Screening on Behalf of a Patient with Medicare and without Health Insurance from Those Who Responded

Primary care physician number and insurance status		Type of priceprovided	Actual price provided	Price reflective of consumers' completecost estimates (Y/N)?[a]	Examples of responses from representatives[b]
1.	Medicare	Billed charge	$75 for an office visit for a person without insurance	N – Does not reflect negotiated rates, include associated fees, or identify out-of-pocket costs	Price is different for everyone. Patient would need to come in for office visit and then the physician would decide on a test.
2.	Medicare	Billed charge, Medicare deductible and co-payment	$125 for an office visit, $250 to $500 quarterly, and 20% of the office visit (about $25)	N – Does not include associated fees	Not sure what the lab would charge.
3.	Medicare	Range of billed charges	$100 to $200 for office visit for a person without insurance	N – Does not reflect negotiated rates, include associated fees, or identify out-of-pocket costs	There would be other tests that would need to happen depending upon a visit with the physician.
4.	Medicare	Billed charges	Physician fee is $85, blood draw is $25	N – Does not reflect negotiated rates or identify out-of-pocket costs	Unsure of what Medicare would cover.
5.	Medicare	None	N/A	N/A	Did not know what Medicare covers or the charge amount. The lab services are also an additional charge and are billed separately.
6.	Medicare	None	N/A	N/A	The price varies based on the office visit and the diagnosis and whatever Medicare would pay. Lab work would also cost extra.

Primary care physician number and insurance status		Type of priceprovided	Actual price provided	Price reflective of consumers' completecost estimates (Y/N)?[a]	Examples of responses from representatives[b]
7.	Medicare	Billed charge	$90 to see a physician	N – Does not reflect negotiated rates, include associated fees, or identify out-of-pocket costs	Requested the name of the specific test as it would be ordered from the physician. They needed to know what services the physician would order to determine the price.
8.	Medicare	Billed charge	$33 for nurse's visit, $8 for glucose test	N – Does not reflect negotiated rates or identify out-of-pocket costs	Unsure of the price Medicare would charge.
9.	Medicare	None	N/A	N/A	Respondent had no idea how much it would cost and said they are not taking new Medicare patients anyway.
10.	Uninsured	Billed charges	$159 to see a physician	N – Does not include associated fees[c]	Have to be seen by a physician before determining costs. For lab tests, the price depends because some tests are done by the lab and some are given in the office.
11.	Uninsured	Billed charges	$120 to see a physician, $37.40 for a comprehensive metabolic panel, $66 for a 1 hour screen	Y[c]	Have to be seen by a doctor first to determine what services are needed.
12	Uninsured	Billed charges	$241 to see physician, $14 for the glucose test, and $32 for a blood draw	N – Does not include associated fees[c]	Unsure of the lab cost because it is a separate charge. It can range based on what services the patient receives.

Table 6. (Continued)

Primary care physician number and insurance status		Type of priceprovided	Actual price provided	Price reflective of consumers' completecost estimates (Y/N)?[a]	Examples of responses from representatives[b]
13.	Uninsured	Range of billed charges	\$89 - \$150 to see a physician, 30% discount for self-paying patients	N – Does not include associated feesc	Need to be seen by a physician here to determine what lab work would need to be done. A range is provided because it depends on the complexity of the visit.
14.	Uninsured	Billed charges	\$250 for a new patient exam and the test is \$125 including blood work	Y[c]	Did not provide.
15.	Uninsured	Billed charges	\$57 for the test and about \$120 for office visit. There is a 30% discount for the office visit for paying day of.	Y	The price depends on the length of the visit.
16.	Uninsured	Range of co-payment if qualifies for Colorado Indigent Care Program (CICP)d	\$5 - 35	Y	Without being in the CICP program, they could not provide price information.
17.	Uninsured	None	N/A	N/A	Person needs to be an established patient and have a physical every year. Also the physician does not take uninsured patients.

Primary care physician number and insurance status		Type of priceprovided	Actual price provided	Price reflective of consumers' completecost estimates (Y/N)?[a]	Examples of responses from representatives[b]
18.	Uninsured	Range of billed charges and billed charge	$120 for physician's visit and test could range from $100 to $500	N – Does not include associated fees[c]	Blood tests are billed separately. The tests done will depend upon what services the physician orders.

Source: GAO analysis of anonymous phone calls to primary care physicians' offices.

aIn cases where a representative did not mention a negotiated discount for an uninsured patient, we assumed that a negotiated discount was not applicable.

bWhen asked for additional information by a physician representative, we did not provide it in order to help maintain our anonymity.

cAccording to the physician representative we spoke with, the billed charges provided were considered an out-of-pocket cost for an uninsured consumer.

dCICP provides funding to clinics and hospitals for Colorado residents or migrant farm workers who are United States citizens or legal immigrants, who have income and resources combined at or below 250 percent of the Federal Poverty Level, and are not eligible for the Medicaid Program or Child Health Plan Plus.

End Notes

[1] Office of the Actuary, Centers for Medicare and Medicaid Services, *National Health Expenditures Tables*, table 1, accessed November 23, 2010, https://www.cms.gov/NationalHealthExpendData/downloads/tables.pdf.

[2] Many health plans require enrollees to pay a portion of their health care costs up to a certain threshold, known as the deductible. A high deductible health plan is defined by the Internal Revenue Service (IRS) as a health plan with a higher annual deductible than typical health plans and has a maximum limit on the annual deductible and out-of-pocket medical expenses (including copayments but not premiums) that a consumer would pay. For 2011, the IRS set the minimum annual deductible for single coverage in a high deductible health plan at $1,200 and the maximum annual deductible and other out-of-pocket expense at $5,950. IRS Pub. 969, (2011), p. 3.

[3] The Kaiser Family Foundation and Health Research & Educational Trust, *Employer Health Benefits 2010 Annual Survey* (2010).

[4] In this report, we generally refer to "price" as information that is made available to the public by, for example, an insurer or state price transparency initiative. We generally refer to "cost" as a type of price information that is reflective of what a consumer may be expected to pay for a health care service.

[5] For example, to assist decision making, research suggests that health care price transparency is most relevant for consumers who are having services that are nonurgent, such as a knee replacement, or not complex, such as a colonoscopy. See, for example, Paul Ginsburg. "Shopping for Price in Medical Care," *Health Affairs*, vol. 26, no. 2 (2007).

[6] In addition to identifying consumers' out-of-pocket costs, research suggests that price information should also be actionable, easy to understand, easily available, timely, credible, and be paired with quality information. See, for example, Quality Alliance Steering Committee, *Recommendations for Reporting Cost and Price Information to Consumers*, accessed August 18, 2010, www.healthqualityalliance.org/.../CostPrice%20 Recommendations_Final.pdf.

[7] Specifically, CMS's online Medicare Plan Finder tool enables consumers to compare both the prices of prescription drugs and Medicare Part D prescription drug coverage plans. Another CMS initiative, entitled Health Care Consumer Initiatives, provides price information based on what Medicare pays for common health care services at the county or other geographic areas, state, and national levels. Additionally, in June 2011, CMS proposed rules to allow organizations that meet certain qualifications to access Medicare claims data in an effort to help consumers and employers select high-quality, low-price health care providers. 76 Fed. Reg. 33567 (June 8, 2011).

[8] National Conference of State Legislatures, *State Legislation Relating to Transparency and Disclosure of Health and Hospital Charges* (Updated December 2010), accessed June 9, 2011, http://www.ncsl.org/default.aspx?tabid=14512. GAO did not independently verify the laws reviewed in this study. State price transparency legislation makes price information available to consumers through various forms, such as requiring hospitals to make information available upon request or requiring hospitals to submit price information to a state agency that makes the information publicly available.

[9] America's Health Insurance Plans, *Health Care Provider Financial Information: State Reporting Requirements* (January 2011).

[10] PPACA, § 1001, 124 Stat. 119, 130-8, amended by § 10101(f), 124 Stat. 119, 885-7 (codified at 42 U.S.C. § 300gg-18).

[11] PPACA, § 1311, 124 Stat. 119, 173-181, amended by § 10104(f), 124 Stat. 119, 900-01 (codified at 42 U.S.C. § 18031(e)(3)(C)). States have flexibility in designing their Exchanges to meet local needs, as long as the health insurance plans offered meet minimum certification standards established by the federal government. The federal government is exploring ways to partner on an Exchange with states that will not be certified by January 1, 2014.

[12] PPACA, § 10104(f), 124 Stat. 119, 900-01 (codified at 42 U.S.C. § 18031(e)(3)(C)). To implement these Exchanges, HHS has issued guidance and has begun the rulemaking process. For example, in July 2011, CMS issued proposed rules that include requirements that states must meet if they elect to establish and operate an Exchange and requirements that health insurance plans must meet to participate in the Exchanges, among other things. For more information, see 76 Fed. Reg. 41,866 (July 15, 2011) and 76 Fed. Reg. 41930 (July 15, 2011). Additionally, according to CMS officials, healthcare.gov also provides cost sharing information such as deductible and out-of-pocket costs for consumers.

[13] We identified relevant literature by searching on an Internet search engine using the term "health care price transparency" in conjunction with the following terms: "legal barriers," "regulatory barriers," "factors," "antitrust laws," "violation of privacy," "proprietary," and "barriers to." Additionally, we searched the Congressional Budget Office's and Congressional Research Service's websites, as well as previous work conducted by GAO.

[14] To identify researchers with subject-matter expertise we reviewed relevant literature and selected researchers who testified before Congress in matters related to price transparency or who authored relevant literature.

[15] Specifically, Colorado requires each licensed hospital to disclose, upon request, the average facility charge to a person seeking care or treatment for a frequently performed inpatient procedure prior to admission for such a procedure. Colo. Rev. Stat. § 6-20-101 (2011). We selected Colorado in part because its law does not specify the manner in which consumers may request price information from hospitals, thus making the state more suitable for requests by telephone.

[16] For the purposes of this study, we are excluding initiatives that are focused solely on providing the prices of prescription drugs or insurance plans.

[17] We also reviewed the Office of Personnel Management's (OPM) Federal Employee Health Benefits (FEHB) program. OPM administers this program by setting price transparency expectations, such as a minimum number of health care services to include, for insurance companies that participate in FEHB. Due to the third party relationship of OPM in providing price information to consumers, we do not discuss OPM's price transparency initiative along with the other selected price transparency initiatives. In addition, the federal government has other price transparency initiatives that do not meet our definition of a price transparency initiative, such as HHS's Medicare Plan Finder and healthcare.gov.

[18] In some cases, a statewide initiative is administered by a private third party entity, such as a state hospital association, but the state has a role in its initiation, regulation, or ongoing development of the price transparency initiative. In these cases, we have classified these as "public (state) initiatives" for the purpose of our review.

[19] In our review we identified several types of private sector price transparency initiatives, such as websites that aggregate price information from public sources and companies that contract with employers to provide health care price information for the company's employees.

[20] Some research indicates that uninsured patients rarely pay the full billed charge, and amounts charged may be heavily discounted based on charity care or other reduced payment programs. For example, one source estimates that most hospitals in the United States collect

only 5 percent or less of billed charges from uninsured patients. See, for example, William O. Cleverly, Paula H. Song, and James O. Cleverly, *Essentials of Health Care Finance*, 7th ed. (Sudbury, MA: Jones & Bartlett Learning, 2011). For more information also see, Uwe E. Reinhardt, "The Pricing of U.S. Hospital Services: Chaos Behind a Veil of Secrecy," *Health Affairs*, 25, no. 1 (2006); and Mark Merlis, "Health Care Price Transparency and Price Competition," National Health Policy Forum (Mar. 28, 2007).

[21] PPACA, § 3023, 124 Stat. 119, 399 (codified at 42 U.S.C. § 1395cc-4).

[22] AHRQ is an agency within HHS, whose mission is to improve the quality, safety, efficiency, and effectiveness of health care by using evidence to improve health care, improving health care outcomes through research, and transforming research into practice. AHRQ also sponsors the Healthcare Cost and Utilization Project which is a family of health care databases and related software tools developed through a federalstate-industry partnership to build a multistate health data system for health care research and decision making. These databases include clinical and nonclinical information, such as charges for all patients regardless of payer by various regions and areas in the United States. We did not include this project in our study because it did not meet our definition of a price transparency initiative.

[23] Specifically, these measures are part of AHRQ's Talking Quality program which provides guidance for sponsors of consumer reports on health care quality. The specific measures cited above relate to the Institute of Medicine's six domains of health care quality, which includes patient safety, effectiveness, patient-centeredness, timeliness, efficiency, and equity measures.

[24] For more information on our work on value in health care, see GAO, *Value in Health Care: Key Information for Policymakers to Assess Efforts to Improve Quality While Reducing Costs*, GAO-11-445 (Washington, D.C.: July 26, 2011).

[25] See, for example, E.A. Halm, C. Lee, and M.R. Chassin, "Is Volume Related to Outcome in Health Care? A Systematic Review and Methodologic Critique of the Literature" *Annals of Internal Medicine*, vol. 137, no. 6 (2002).

[26] Exec. Order No. 13,410, 71 Fed. Reg. 51,089 (Aug. 28, 2006). The executive order also directed agencies to improve usage of health information technology, implement programs to measure quality of services, and identify and develop approaches that facilitate high-quality and efficient health care.

[27] National Conference of State Legislatures, *State Legislation Relating to Transparency and Disclosure of Health and Hospital Charges* (Updated December 2010), accessed June 9, 2011, http://www.ncsl.org/default.aspx?tabid=14512.

[28] Colo. Rev. Stat. § 6-20-101 (2011), S.D. Codified Laws § 34-12E-8 (Michie 2010). [29]Me. Rev. Stat. Ann. title 22 § 8712(2) (West 2011), Minn. Stat. § 62J.82 (2011).

[30] See http://healthcarebluebook.com/ and http://www.pricedoc.com/ for more information.

[31] See, for example, Congressional Research Service, *Does Price Transparency Improve Market Efficiency? Implications of Empirical Evidence in Other Markets for the Health Sector*, RL34101 (Apr. 29, 2008); and Paul Ginsburg, "Shopping for Price in Medical Care," *Health Affairs*, vol. 26, no. 2 (2007).

[32] See, for example, The Commonwealth Fund Commission on a High Performance Health System, *Data Brief – Health Care Opinion Leaders' Views on the Transparency of Health Care Quality and Price Information in the United States* (New York: The Commonwealth Fund, November 2007).

[33] See for example, Paul Ginsburg, "Shopping for Price in Medical Care," *Health Affairs*, vol. 26, no. 2 (2007).

[34] See appendix I for the information we obtained when contacting selected providers about the price of selected health care services.

[35] For more information, see "The Opportunity of Price Transparency," *Healthcare Financial Management Association* (2007): 4. The Healthcare Financial Management Association is an organization that seeks to provide education, analysis, and guidance, among other things, to health care finance professionals.

[36] For example, officials from one insurance company said one of the contractual obligations with a provider states that the insurer is prohibited from disclosing specific negotiated contract rates to its members, unless such information is provided in an explanation of benefits or through calls placed individually to the insurer's member services department.

[37] Although the insurance officials said that some providers impose contractual obligations that restrict the disclosure of negotiated rates, officials from one insurance company told us that they were able to negotiate their contracts with providers without such contractual obligations by explaining the methodology used to develop and present price information to consumers.

[38] Many states have adopted the Uniform Trade Secrets Act, proposed by the Uniform Law Commissioners, which protects proprietary information. Uniform Law Commission, Trade Secrets Act, accessed July 14, 2011, http://www.nccusl.org/Act.aspx?title= Trade%20 Secrets%20Act. States that have not adopted the Uniform Trade Secrets Act may have similar laws that protect proprietary information from being misappropriated.

[39] According to the Department of Justice, the three major federal antitrust laws are the Sherman Antitrust Act, the Clayton Act, and the Federal Trade Commission Act. In addition, many states also have antitrust laws.

[40] However, these insurance officials agreed that antitrust restrictions do not prevent the sharing of negotiated rates and other components of complete cost estimates with their members.

[41] See U.S. Department of Justice and the Federal Trade Commission, *Statements of Antitrust Enforcement Policy in Health Care* (1996). According to FTC and DOJ guidance, providers may act individually to provide price information to a purchaser without concern; however under certain circumstances, if they act collectively it may raise antitrust concerns because it may lead to collusion.

[42] While careful adherence to the guidelines will usually not generate FTC or DOJ enforcement action, both agencies have made clear that each case or business practice requires an analysis of the particular facts and circumstances involved. To the extent that any uncertainty exists, a provider or other entity may take advantage of DOJ's expedited business review procedure or FTC's advisory opinion procedure for guidance in order to alleviate antitrust concerns.

[43] New Hampshire's and Massachusetts' claims data include all payments for that service contributed by private health insurance plans and their members, as well as payments from self-insured plans for state government employees and their members.

[44] The selected price transparency initiatives use different terms to refer to what we describe as the health care "services" for which consumers can look up price information.

[45] In some cases, the state law specified the number or types of services made available by the price transparency initiative. See, e.g., Cal. Health & Safety Code § 1339.56(a) (2008), Fla. Stat. Ann. § 408.05(3)(k)(4) (West 2011).

[46] Wisconsin's price transparency website, called PricePoint, has served as a model for other states. Since its launch, WHA has been hired by at least 16 states to develop PricePoint websites for their initiatives.

[47] See Cal. Health & Safety Code §§ 1339.56(c) (2008), Fla. Stat. Ann § 408.05 (3)(k)(4) (West 2011). Florida's initiative provides a disclaimer that patients rarely are required to pay billed charges without any discounts and this type of price information may not be the most meaningful indicator of what the consumer can be expected to pay. Similarly, California's initiative acknowledges that the charges do not reflect how much the hospital is typically paid for a service because the discounts have not been applied.

[48] Health care claims data must be submitted to a state agency and such information was then added to the state's price transparency initiative. See Mass Regs. Code tit. 129 § 2.05(3) (2009).

[49] At the same time, CMS officials described reliance on Medicare payment data as a weakness of their initiative because consumers do not know how to understand and use that price data.

[50] See N.H. Rev. Stat. Ann. §§ 420-G:11, 420-G:11-a (2011). APCD is a database of payment reimbursement records to providers that may include claims from private insurance company payers and their members and public payers (Medicare and Medicaid). According to the APCD Council, as of November 2010, 13 states, including Massachusetts, are using or in the process of developing APCDs.

[51] Although presenting prices as ranges, rather than single point estimates, may be useful for avoiding proprietary concerns, ranges may also be so broad that they lose the utility for meeting consumers' needs to compare prices and anticipate health care costs.

[52] These nonprice data, such as the frequency or quality of a provider in performing a procedure, is often gathered from national sources, such as WebMD, CMS, and AHRQ, or directly from providers' data submissions, such as data submitted to state agencies, which may vary based on the states' reporting requirements.

[53] Since New Hampshire uses claims data over a year old, officials adjust the claims' prices across the board with a 5 percent increase for every year to account for an estimated annual rate of inflation in medical costs.

[54] Fla. Stat. Ann § 408.061(c) (West 2011).

[55] Furthermore, although Massachusetts has access to claims data that in some cases provide all associated costs, such as physician fees, for a specific health care service, officials there said that they currently lack the technical capability to identify from the claims data which hospital and physician fees should be linked. They noted that insurance plans are not consistent in how they report physician fees in the claims data.

[56] Anthem officials said that they are exploring the possibility of developing an out-of-pocket cost calculator for their consumer initiative.

End Notes for Appendix I

[1] We selected a health care market in Colorado because this state requires certain providers to respond to consumers' requests for price information, but does not restrict how consumers may request such information. For more information, see Colo. Rev. Stat. § 6-20-101 (2011). We did not evaluate the effectiveness of the law. We specifically selected the Denver health care market, as defined by a hospital referral region, because it was the health care market in Colorado with the most hospitals with zip codes in Colorado. A hospital referral region, as defined by the Dartmouth Atlas of Health Care, represents a regional health care market. Furthermore, we determined that the Denver health care market did not

have any characteristics that would make it particularly unique compared to other health care markets in the United States.

[2] For purposes of this study, we contacted selected providers using contact information from the Centers for Medicare and Medicaid Services' (CMS) Hospital Compare database (for hospitals) and the National Provider Identifier Registry (for primary care physicians). We excluded hospitals and physicians with addresses located outside of Denver, Colorado, for the purposes of this study. We contacted 19 hospitals because there were only 19 hospitals in the Denver, Colorado, hospital referral region that provided knee replacement surgery, according to CMS's Hospital Compare database. For primary care physicians, we randomly selected a nonrepresentative group of 20 physicians with a specialty such as internal medicine, family medicine, and general practice to be a comparable sample size to that of the hospitals.

[3] According to the American Medical Association, CPT is a medical nomenclature used to report medical procedures and services under public and private insurance programs.

[4] According to Hospital Compare, CMS's quality and price transparency initiative, the median Medicare payment to hospitals within 25 miles of Denver, Colorado, for a major joint replacement or reattachment of a lower extremity without major complications or comorbidities ranges from $446 to $18,668. According to CMS officials, there may be a wide range of median Medicare payments to hospitals for this health care service because the data provided in Hospital Compare include cases in which Medicare was only responsible for a portion of the payment. Because these cases do not reflect the full amount paid for a service, CMS officials stated that they plan to remove these cases from the data in October 2011.

[5] According to Medicare.gov, Medicare patients may receive two free diabetes screening tests per year and they generally have to pay 20 percent of the Medicare-approved amount for the doctor's visit.

In: Health Care in the United States
Editor: Leone Giangiulio
ISBN: 978-1-62618-413-8

Chapter 2

PRIVATE HEALTH INSURANCE: ESTIMATES OF INDIVIDUALS WITH PRE-EXISTING CONDITIONS RANGE FROM 36 MILLION TO 122 MILLION*

United States Government Accountability Office

WHY GAO DID THIS STUDY

Individuals who buy coverage directly from a health insurer are often denied coverage due to a pre-existing condition during a process called medical underwriting, which assesses an applicant's health status and other risk factors. Beginning January 1, 2014, the Patient Protection and Affordable Care Act (PPACA) prohibits health insurers in the individual market from denying coverage, increasing premiums, or restricting benefits because of a pre-existing condition. GAO was asked to examine the effect of this provision on adults who are 19- 64 years old. GAO examined (1) the most common medical conditions that would cause an insurance company to restrict or deny insurance coverage for adults and the average annual costs associated with these conditions, (2) estimates of the number of adults with pre-existing

---

* This is an edited, reformatted and augmented version of United States Government Accountability Office, Publication No. GAO-12-439, dated March 2012.

conditions, and (3) the geographic and demographic profile of adults with pre-existing conditions.

To address these three issues, GAO (1) identified four recent studies that narrowly or more broadly identified five lists of conditions likely to result in restricted coverage in the individual insurance market and (2) used the 2009 Medical Expenditure Panel Survey to generate five separate estimates, referred to as estimates 1 through 5. There is no commonly accepted list of pre-existing conditions because each insurer determines the conditions it will use for medical underwriting. We also contacted state insurance department officials in all 50 states and the District of Columbia to confirm information about state insurance protections that currently limit or prohibit medical underwriting.

WHAT GAO FOUND

Hypertension was the most commonly reported medical condition among adults that could result in a health insurer denying coverage, requiring higher-thanaverage premiums, or restricting coverage. GAO's analysis found that about 33.2 million adults age 19-64 years old, or about 18 percent, reported hypertension in 2009. Individuals with hypertension reported average annual expenditures related to treating the condition of $650, but maximum reported expenditures were $61,540. Mental health disorders and diabetes were the second and third most commonly reported conditions among adults. Cancer was the condition with the highest average annual treatment expenditures—about $9,000.

Depending on the list of conditions used to define pre-existing conditions in each of the five estimates, GAO found that between 36 million and 122 million adults reported medical conditions that could result in a health insurer restricting coverage. This represents between 20 and 66 percent of the adult population, with a midpoint estimate of about 32 percent. The differences among the estimates can be attributed to the number and type of conditions included in the different lists of pre-existing conditions. For example, estimate 1, which is the lowest estimate, includes adults reporting that they had ever been told they had 1 or more of 8 conditions. Estimate 3, the midpoint estimate, includes any individual reporting they had one of over 60 conditions. Estimate 5, the highest estimate, includes any individual reporting a chronic condition in 2009.

The estimated number of adults with pre-existing conditions varies by state, but most individuals, 88-89 percent depending on the list of pre-existing conditions included, live in states that do not report having insurance protections similar to those in PPACA. Compared to others, adults with pre-existing conditions spend thousands of dollars more annually on health care, but pre-existing conditions are common across all family income levels.

The Department of Health and Human Services reviewed a draft of this report and had no substantive or technical comments.

ABBREVIATIONS

AHRQ	Agency for Healthcare Research and Quality
FPL	federal poverty level
HCERA	Health Care and Education Reconciliation Act of 2010
HHS	Department of Health and Human Services
HIPAA	Health Insurance Portability and Accountability Act of 1998
ICD-9-CM	International Classification of Diseases, Ninth Edition, Clinical Modification
MEPS	Medical Expenditure Panel Survey
PCIP	Pre-Existing Condition Insurance Plan
PPACA	Patient Protection and Affordable Care Act

March 27, 2012
Congressional Requesters

Americans obtain health insurance coverage through a variety of private and public sources, but a majority—67 percent of adults as of 2010—rely on private insurance, most through employer-sponsored group coverage. Another 16 percent of adults in 2010 had coverage through public programs, such as Medicare and Medicaid, and about 22 percent were uninsured.[1,2] While group health plans and health insurers offering group coverage may not condition eligibility based on an individual's health status, such protections generally do not exist for individuals attempting to purchase coverage directly through the private individual market, which accounted for about 14.6 million adults aged 18-64 years old in 2010.[3] In addition, individuals are at risk of losing the protections of employer-sponsored group coverage if they become unemployed or retire before eligibility for Medicare begins at age 65 and they have a break in health coverage. With certain exceptions, such individuals and any other individual attempting to purchase coverage in the private individual market can have coverage denied, offered at a higher-than-average premium, or offered with a rider that excludes coverage of a pre-existing condition. A pre-existing condition is a health condition that exists before someone applies for or enrolls in a new health insurance policy. Each insurer develops its own list of pre-existing conditions that influences to whom and under what terms it offers coverage. Pre-existing conditions can be conditions that an individual is currently being treated for (such as heart disease) or past health problems (such as cancer in remission).

With the enactment of the Patient Protection and Affordable Care Act (PPACA) in March 2010, enrollment in private health insurance could expand significantly, particularly for individuals and families that do not have access to group coverage through their employer.[4] PPACA provisions that could expand such coverage include income-based subsidies to make coverage more affordable for certain individuals, penalties for individuals not obtaining coverage, and new insurance requirements to increase access to coverage, particularly for individuals with pre-existing conditions. Specifically, beginning January 1, 2014, health insurers in the individual market will be prohibited from denying coverage, increasing premiums, or restricting benefits because of a preexisting condition.[5]

To better understand the potential impact of PPACA, you asked us to examine the demographics of adults with pre-existing conditions. In this report, we examine: (1) the most common medical conditions that would cause an insurance company to restrict or deny insurance coverage for adults and the average annual costs associated with these conditions, estimates of the number of adults with pre-existing conditions, and the geographic and demographic profile of adults with pre-existing conditions. We define adults as age 19-64 years old in this report because a PPACA provision prohibiting insurers from denying coverage or restricting benefits because of a pre-existing condition for individuals under the age of 19 became effective September 23, 2010, and Medicare covers individuals 65 and older.

To address these three issues, we identified several recent studies that listed conditions considered likely to result in restricted coverage in the individual insurance market and then used the 2009 Medical Expenditure Panel Survey (MEPS) to analyze the conditions listed in each study in order to develop estimates of (1) the number of adults reporting and costs associated with treating specific pre-existing conditions, (2) size of the total affected adult population with pre-existing conditions, and (3) their geographic and demographic characteristics. MEPS is a commonly used, nationally representative, and publicly available panel survey of Americans; 2009 was the most recent year data were available.[6] It includes information on medical conditions and the costs associated with those medical conditions, both self-reported and from a review of medical events.[7]

We identified four recent studies that used different lists of pre-existing conditions to develop five estimates of the number of affected individuals. Each of these studies identified a set of conditions that would cause an insurance company to deny health insurance coverage, offer coverage at a higher-than-average premium, or offer coverage with restrictions. The sets of conditions run the continuum from narrow (having one of eight conditions that would qualify an individual for participation in a high-risk pool) to broad (reporting any condition considered chronic).[8,9]

Each insurer separately determines which conditions will result in restricted coverage in the individual insurance market, so lists of conditions may not be consistent from insurer to insurer.

As shown in table 1, there were important differences across the four studies, including the conditions and time frames considered, the populations that the estimates were developed for (e.g., children and adults under age 65, or solely the uninsured), the data sources used to develop the estimates, and whether the study included only individuals treated for a condition during a given year or individuals ever diagnosed with a condition.

We used the set of conditions developed for each study to generate estimates of adults with pre-existing conditions using a consistent data source (2009 MEPS) and population (19-64 year olds not enrolled in Medicare). We assigned each condition list an estimate number from 1 to 5 in order to more readily identify which set of study conditions each estimate is based on. For example, the condition list in the study authored by Harold Pollack is referred to as estimate 1.

To describe the geographic and demographic profile of adults with pre-existing conditions, we further analyzed data on the low, midpoint, and high estimates of adults with pre-existing conditions.

To enable us to develop estimates of individuals with pre-existing conditions living in states reporting insurance protections similar to those that will be offered under PPACA in 2014, we updated information on state insurance protections previously reported by the Kaiser Family Foundation by contacting state insurance department officials in all 50 states and the District of Columbia. Appendix I contains a full description of our scope and methodology.

Table 1. Information on Studies Used to Estimate the Number of Adults with Pre-existing Conditions

	Study author	Population studied	Estimated number of population studied with pre-existing conditions	Included conditions respondent reported as occurring during the survey year	Included conditions respondent reported ever being diagnosed with	Data source	Data year
Estimate 1	Harold Pollack[a]	Uninsured of any age	4.1 million	No	Yes	National Health and Nutrition Examination Survey[b]	2005/2006
Estimate 2[c]	Department of Health and Human Services[c]	Age 0-64	50 million	Yes	Yes	Medical Expenditure Panel Survey (MEPS)[d]	2008
Estimate 3	Families USA[e]	Age 0-64	57.2 million	Yes	No	MEPS	2007
Estimate 4[c]	Department of Health and Human Services[c]	Age 0-64	129 million	Yes	Yes	MEPS	2008
Estimate 5	GAO[f]	Uninsured of any age in 34 states with high-risk health insurance pools	4.0 million	Yes	No	MEPS	2006

Source: GAO analysis.

Note: High-risk pools are designed for individuals who cannot obtain insurance in the individual market because of a pre-existing condition. Therefore, estimates of individuals potentially eligible for high-risk pools should be roughly equivalent to those of individuals with pre-existing conditions.

[a]H. Pollack, "High-Risk Pools for the Sick and Uninsured under Health Reform: Too Little and Thus Too Late," *Journal of General Internal Medicine*, published online Sept. 2, 2010.

[b]The National Health and Nutrition Examination Survey is sponsored by the Centers for Disease Control and Prevention, an agency within the Department of Health and Human Services (HHS).

[c]Department of Health and Human Services, "At Risk: Pre-Existing Conditions Could Affect 1 in 2 Americans: 129 Million People Could Be Denied Affordable Coverage without Health Reform" (Washington, D.C.: January 2011). This study produced two separate estimates of individuals with pre-existing conditions based on two different condition lists.

[d]The Medical Expenditure Panel Survey is sponsored by the Agency for Healthcare Research and Quality, an agency within HHS.

[e]Families USA, "Health Reform: Help for Americans with Pre-Existing Conditions" (Washington, D.C.: May 2010).

[f]GAO, *Health Insurance: Enrollment, Benefits, Funding, and Other Characteristics of State High-Risk Health Insurance Pools*, GAO-09-730R (Washington, D.C.: July 22, 2009).

To assess the reliability of the MEPS data, we reviewed the relevant documentation, compared our estimates to other published results, and interviewed an official at the Agency for Healthcare Research and Quality (AHRQ), the federal agency responsible for the MEPS. We determined the data are sufficiently reliable for the purposes of our report.

We conducted this performance audit from July 2011 to March 2012 in accordance with generally accepted government auditing standards. Those standards require that we plan and perform the audit to obtain sufficient, appropriate evidence to provide a reasonable basis for our findings and conclusions based on our audit objectives. We believe that the evidence obtained provides a reasonable basis for our findings and conclusions based on our audit objectives.

BACKGROUND

Individuals who buy coverage directly from a health insurer are often denied coverage due to a pre-existing condition. We previously reported that in the first quarter of 2010, 19 percent of applicants in the individual market were denied enrollment and a quarter of insurers had denial rates of 40 percent or higher.[10] Similarly, a study by America's Health Insurance Plans reported that in 2008, 15 percent of individual insurance applications for adults age 18 through 64 that went through medical underwriting were denied coverage.[11] Medical underwriting is the process conducted by insurers to assess an applicant's health status and other risk factors to determine whether and on what terms to offer coverage to applicants.

The Health Insurance Portability and Accountability Act of 1996 (HIPAA) established consumer protections on access, portability, and renewability of health insurance coverage. 12 With respect to individuals leaving group coverage and applying for coverage in the individual market, HIPAA prohibited health insurers from denying coverage to or imposing any preexisting condition exclusion on individuals who

- have had at least 18 months of prior creditable coverage with no break of more than 63 days;
- have exhausted any available continuation coverage;
- are uninsured and are not eligible for other group coverage, Medicare, or Medicaid; and

- did not lose group coverage because of the nonpayment of premiums or fraud.[13]

Unless the practice is prohibited by state law, individuals who do not meet these HIPAA eligibility criteria can be denied insurance coverage in the individual market due to a pre-existing condition. Additionally, insurers in the individual market can accept both HIPAA-eligible and noneligible applicants but offer coverage at a premium that is higher than the standard rate based on the presence of a pre-existing condition. A medical condition reported by an individual is considered a pre-existing condition by the insurer if it exists at the time the individual applies for coverage or if an individual was treated for or diagnosed with the condition in the past.

States, which have the responsibility for regulating private insurance, have in some instances required protections for individuals with preexisting conditions. State protections include the following:

- Guaranteed issue requirements prohibit the denial of coverage to individuals based on pre-existing conditions. In some states, all products must be guaranteed issue, while in other states guaranteed issue requirements are only applicable to some products or to some individuals, for instance individuals with 12 months of continuous coverage, or to some standard products, such as a basic health plan.
- An insurer of last resort law requires one insurer in the state to issue products to individuals regardless of pre-existing conditions.
- Rating restrictions prohibit insurers in the individual market from adjusting an individual's health insurance premiums based on an individual's health status.
- Two types of rating restrictions are pure community rating and adjusted community rating. Under the former, insurers may not adjust premiums due to health status, age, or gender; under the latter, they may adjust premiums according to characteristics such as gender or age, depending on the state.
- Rate bands limit the extent to which premiums can vary based on an individual's health status, for example, to a certain percentage of the average premium.
- Limitations on the number of years a health insurer can look back at an individual's health history when making its determination as to whether and at what price to offer coverage.

- High-risk health insurance pools that provide coverage to individuals whose health status, including the presence of pre-existing conditions, limits their access to coverage in the private individual health insurance market.[14] High-risk insurance pools—typically publicly subsidized, state-run nonprofit associations—often contract with a private health insurer to administer the pool and offer a range of health plan options.

Until 2014, PPACA requires that individuals who have pre-existing conditions and have been uninsured for 6 months be offered the opportunity to enroll in a temporary national high-risk pool program, known as the Pre-Existing Condition Insurance Plan (PCIP).[15] PCIP will close at the end of 2013, which is when PPACA will begin to require insurers to accept every individual who applies for coverage, regardless of factors related to health status. States were given the option of running their own PCIP with federal funding, or allowing the Department of Health and Human Services (HHS) to administer the PCIP in their state. Twenty-seven states elected to administer a PCIP for their residents, while 23 states and the District of Columbia opted to allow HHS to administer their PCIPs. Despite similar goals, PCIP and state high-risk pools are separate entities and differ from one another in certain ways.[16]

Beginning in 2014, PPACA prohibits insurers in the private individual market from denying coverage, charging higher-than-average premiums, or restricting coverage to individuals based on the individual's health status. PPACA will, therefore, make guaranteed issue and adjusted community rating national requirements.

Hypertension, Mental Health Disorders, and Diabetes Were the Most Commonly Reported Conditions among Adults, with Average Annual Expenditures for Cancer Nearly $9,000

Hypertension was the most commonly reported medical condition among adults during 2009 that could result in a health insurer denying coverage, requiring higher-than-average premiums, or restricting coverage with an exclusionary rider.[17]

Table 2. Estimates of Adults (Age 19-64) Reporting Specified Conditions and Average Expenditures Associated with Each Condition for Those with Any Expenditures, 2009

	Estimate (number)	Range based on 95 percent confidence interval	Percentage estimate	Percentage range based on 95 percent confidence interval	Average annual expenditures related to condition (dollars)	Maximum expenditures related to condition (dollars)
Total population	184,648,891	176,372,785 – 192,924,998	100.0%	—	—	—
Hypertension	33,207,272	31,145,377 – 35,269,167	18.0	17.2 – 18.8	$650	$61,540
Mental health disorders[a]	18,995,244	17,516,845 – 20,473,642	10.3	9.7 – 10.9	$1,757	$98,058
Diabetes	11,899,811	11,007,195 – 12,792,427	6.4	6.0 – 6.9	$1,782	$66,007
Asthma	10,047,807	9,177,963 – 10,917,652	5.4	5.0 – 5.9	$1,234	$63,003
Arthritis[b]	9,518,122	8,513,144 – 10,523,099	5.2	4.7 – 5.7	$1,875	$78,617
Chronic obstructive pulmonary disease	9,091,824	8,305,480 – 9,878,167	4.9	4.5 – 5.3	$1,423[c]	$172,583
Cancer (excluding skin)	4,150,263	3,588,601 – 4,711,924	2.3	2.0 – 2.5	$8,955	$294,473
Rheumatoid arthritis	3,041,838	2,621,846 – 3,461,831	1.7	1.4 – 1.9	$2,691	$39,228
Heart attack (myocardial infarction)	2,056,226	1,678,883 – 2,433,568	1.1	0.9 – 1.3	$4,013	$53,666
Stroke	1,291,310	1,008,677 – 1,573,943	0.7	0.6 – 0.9	$6,224[c]	$109,324

Source: GAO analysis of Medical Expenditure Panel Survey (MEPS).

Notes: Adults are defined as individuals age 19-64. Adults with Medicare coverage were excluded. Estimates are of individuals who reported that these conditions were the cause of a medical event, the reason for a disability day, or bothered a respondent during 2009. Estimates were generated only for conditions with a cell size of more than 100. Expenditure information is reported only for those with expenditures greater than $0 and includes expenditures from all sources for hospital inpatient stays, emergency room visits, outpatient department visits, office-based medical provider visits, and prescribed medicines. Expenditure information does not include amounts for dental expenses and other medical expenses, such as durable and nondurable supplies, medical equipment, eyeglasses, and ambulance services because these items could not be linked to specific conditions. We also did not include expenditures for home health care.

[a]Mental health disorders are defined as mood and psychotic disorders, which include conditions such as depression, bipolar disorder, and schizophrenia.

[b]Arthritis includes osteoarthritis, rheumatoid arthritis, and infective arthritis.

[c]The relative standard error is greater than or equal to 30 percent. Relative standard error is the proportion of the standard error divided by the estimate itself.

Our analysis of MEPS data found that about 33.2 million adults age 19-64 years old, or about 18 percent, reported hypertension in 2009. Individuals with hypertension reported average annual expenditures of $650 related to treating the condition, though the maximum expenditures reported were $61,540.[18] (See table 2.)

Mental health disorders and diabetes were the second and third most commonly reported medical conditions by adults age 19-64 years old.[19] About 19.0 million adults, or 10.3 percent, reported mental health disorders, and about 11.9 million adults, or about 6.4 percent, reported diabetes. Average annual expenditures for these conditions were $1,757 for mental health disorders and $1,782 for diabetes. Cancer was the condition with the highest average annual treatment expenditures, nearly $9,000 per adult. Individuals may have multiple medical conditions, which would increase their total expenditures.

The number of adults reporting specific conditions in any given year does not include all adults who may have had that condition in the past. For instance, there are many individuals who may have had cancer in the past who would not report cancer in a given year.

Therefore, the number of adults who have ever had cancer is higher than the approximately 4.2 million reporting cancer in 2009. About 11 million adults, or 6.0 percent, reported ever being told by a health professional that they had cancer. Health insurers commonly look at both current medical conditions and conditions an individual was treated for or diagnosed with in the past when making a decision whether and at what price to offer health insurance coverage.

Between 36 and 122 Million Adults in 2009 Reported Pre-Existing Conditions, Depending on the Conditions Included in the Estimates

Depending on the list of conditions used to define pre-existing conditions in each of five estimates, we found that between 36 million and 122 million adults (age 19-64) reported having medical conditions in 2009 that could result in a health insurer denying coverage, requiring higherthan-average premiums, or restricting coverage with an exclusionary rider (see fig. 1).

This represents from 20 to 66 percent of the adult population, with a midpoint estimate of 32 percent.

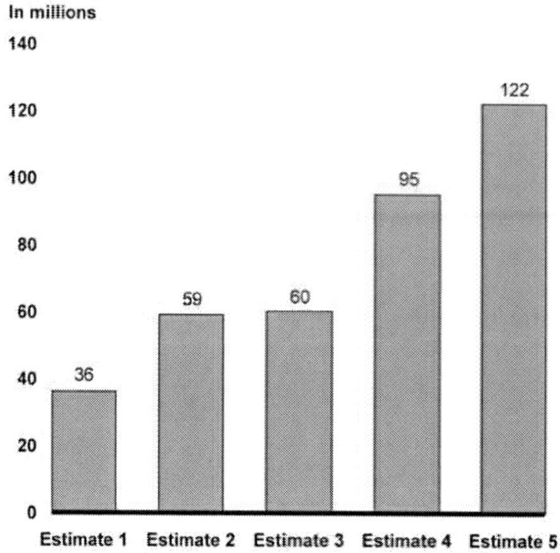

Source: GAO analysis of 2009 Medical Expenditure Panel Survey (MEPS).

Notes: Information on the conditions included in each estimate is detailed in appendix I. Estimate 1 is based on the methodology in Harold Pollack's article "High-Risk Pools for the Sick and Uninsured Under Health Reform: Too Little and Thus Too Late," in the *Journal of General Internal Medicine* (published online on September 2, 2010). Estimates 2 and 4 are based on the methodologies in the Department of Health and Human Services report "At Risk: Pre-Existing Conditions Could Affect 1 in 2 Americans: 129 Million People Could Be Denied Affordable Coverage without Health Reform" (Washington, D.C.: January 2011). Estimate 3 is based on the methodology in the Families USA report "Health Reform: Help for Americans with Pre-Existing Conditions," published in May 2010. Estimate 5 is based on the methodology used in the GAO report *Health Insurance: Enrollment, Benefits, Funding, and Other Characteristics of State High-Risk Health Insurance Pools*, GAO-09-730R (Washington, D.C.: July 22, 2009). The 95 percent confidence intervals for estimates in this figure are within +/- 1 percent of the estimates themselves.

Figure 1. Estimates of Adults (Age 19-64) with Pre-Existing Medical Conditions, 2009.

The differences among the estimates can be attributed to the number and type of conditions included in the different lists of pre-existing conditions. For example, estimate 1, which is the lowest estimate, includes adults reporting that they had ever been told they had 1 or more of 8 conditions. All 8 conditions were designated as priority conditions by AHRQ because of the conditions' prevalence, expense, or relevance to policy.[20]

Estimate 3, the midpoint estimate, includes any individual who had one of over 60 conditions commonly used to determine eligibility in state high-risk pools. Estimate 5, the highest estimate, includes any individual reporting they had experienced any condition considered chronic during 2009.[21] The list of chronic conditions used for this estimate included 417 separate conditions. See appendix I for information on the list of conditions included in each estimate.

PRE-EXISTING CONDITIONS ARE COMMON ACROSS STATES AND DEMOGRAPHIC GROUPS, BUT PREVALENCE IS HIGHER FOR CERTAIN POPULATIONS

The number of adults with pre-existing conditions varies by state, but most individuals with pre-existing conditions live in states that report not having insurance protections similar to PPACA. Certain groups had higher rates of pre-existing conditions than others, including women, whites, and those with public insurance. Compared to others, adults with pre-existing conditions spend thousands of dollars more annually on health care, but pre-existing conditions are common across all family income levels.

The Number of Adults with Pre-Existing Conditions Varies by State, but Most Adults with Pre-Existing Conditions Live in States That Report Not Having Insurance Protections Similar to PPACA

We found that the percentage of adults with pre-existing conditions varies among states. We analyzed data from the 35 states where MEPS generated a reliable estimate.[22] Our low estimate (estimate 1) ranged from 17 percent in New York and New Jersey to 25 percent in Ohio. For the midpoint estimate (estimate 3), the range was from 27 percent in Florida to 47 percent in Kentucky. For the high estimate (estimate 5), the range was from 58 percent in Georgia to 75 percent in Kentucky and Massachusetts. (See table 3). For population estimates for the 35 states, see appendix II.

Table 3. Percent of Adults (Age 19-64) with Pre-Existing Conditions across States, Low, Midpoint, or High Estimate, 2009

State	Low: estimate 1	Midpoint: estimate 3	High: estimate 5
All adults	20	32	66
Alabama	—	—	69
Alaska	—	—	—
Arizona	—	33	65
Arkansas	—	—	66
California	18	29	60
Colorado	—	—	68
Connecticut	—	—	71
Delaware	—	—	—
District of Columbia	—	—	—
Florida	18	27	60
Georgia	21	32	58
Hawaii	—	—	66
Idaho	—	—	—
Illinois	18	33	68
Indiana	—	36	70
Iowa	—	—	74
Kansas	—	—	67
Kentucky	—	47	75
Louisiana	—	—	72
Maine	—	—	—
Maryland	—	—	63
Massachusetts	—	35	75
Michigan	21	41	74
Minnesota	—	—	64
Mississippi	—	—	74
Missouri	—	36	70
Montana	—	—	—
Nebraska	—	—	—
Nevada	—	—	—
New Hampshire	—	—	—
New Jersey	17	30	71
New Mexico	—	—	—
New York	17	31	64
North Carolina	21	32	63
North Dakota	—	—	—

State	Low: estimate 1	Midpoint: estimate 3	High: estimate 5
Ohio	25	35	69
Oklahoma	—	—	61
Oregon	—	—	66
Pennsylvania	20	34	69
Rhode Island	—	—	—
South Carolina	—	—	60
South Dakota	—	—	—
Tennessee	—	30	62
Texas	18	30	63
Utah	—	—	68
Vermont	—	—	—
Virginia	19	30	63
Washington	—	30	71
West Virginia	—	—	—
Wisconsin	—	—	64
Wyoming	—	—	—

Source: GAO analysis of 2009 Medical Expenditure Panel Survey (MEPS).

Notes: Estimate 1 is based on the methodology in Harold Pollack's article "High-Risk Pools for the Sick and Uninsured Under Health Reform: Too Little and Thus Too Late," in the *Journal of General Internal Medicine* (published online on September 2, 2010). Estimate 3 is based on the methodology in the Families USA report "Health Reform: Help for Americans with Pre-Existing Conditions," published in May 2010. Estimate 5 is based on the methodology used in the GAO report *Health Insurance: Enrollment, Benefits, Funding, and Other Characteristics of State High-Risk Health Insurance Pools*, GAO-09-730R (Washington, D.C.: July 22, 2009). The 95 percent confidence intervals for estimates in this table are within +/- 3 percent of the estimates themselves. Due to insufficient sample sizes, MEPS data could not be used to provide any estimates for 15 states and the District of Columbia. Dashes in the table indicate that the sample size was not sufficient to produce an estimate.

We estimate that 88-89 percent of adults with pre-existing conditions live in states without insurance protections similar to the PPACA provisions, which will become effective in 2014. We classified states as having protections similar to PPACA if the state reported having (1) a guaranteed issue requirement for some or all products in the individual insurance market and (2) pure or adjusted community rating.[23] The only five states reporting such protections are Maine, Massachusetts, New Jersey, New York, and Vermont.

While the majority of states do not offer protections similar to what will be required nationally in 2014, many states do offer some protection to individuals with pre-existing conditions. Insurance department officials in 12 states reported having a guaranteed issue requirement for some or all products in the individual insurance market. Eight states reported either pure or adjusted community rating requirements. Appendix III shows the various state protections for individuals with pre-existing conditions in the 50 states and the District of Columbia.

Pre-Existing Conditions Are More Common among Women, Whites, and Those with Public Insurance

Regardless of the list of conditions used to generate the estimates, we found that more women reported a pre-existing condition than men. Based on the different definitions of pre-existing conditions we used, from 21 to 72 percent of women reported a pre-existing condition in 2009.[24] From 18 to 59 percent of men reported a pre-existing condition. The midpoint estimate for women and men was 37 percent and 28 percent, respectively. (See fig. 2.)

We found that the prevalence of pre-existing conditions among adults increases with age (see fig. 3). In the 55- to 64-year-old age group, from 43 (low estimate) to 84 percent (high estimate) of adults reported a preexisting condition that would cause an insurance company to deny coverage, offer coverage at a higher-than-average rate, or restrict coverage. In contrast, from 6 percent (low estimate) to 45 percent (high estimate) of 19-24 year olds (the youngest age group) reported a preexisting condition. The midpoint estimate for 55-64 year olds was 48 percent, as compared to a midpoint estimate of 19 percent for 19-24 year olds.

Asian and Pacific Islanders and Hispanics have the lowest reported rates of pre-existing conditions in each estimate, significantly lower than the rate seen across all adults. For example, for the midpoint estimate, 15 percent of Asian and Pacific Islanders reported a pre-existing condition, compared to 32 percent of all adults. In two of three estimates (the low and high estimates), white adults are slightly more likely to report a pre-existing condition than the adult population as a whole. This difference was statistically significant, but the difference was not statistically significant for the midpoint estimate. (See table 4.)

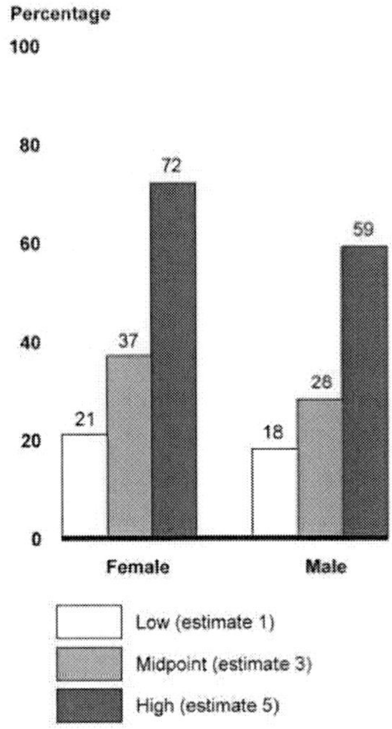

Source: GAO analysis of 2009 Medical Expenditure Panel Survey (MEPS).

Note: Estimate 1 is based on the methodology in Harold Pollack's article "High-Risk Pools for the Sick and Uninsured Under Health Reform: Too Little and Thus Too Late," in the *Journal of General Internal Medicine* (published online on September 2, 2010). Estimate 3 is based on the methodology in the Families USA report "Health Reform: Help for Americans with Pre-Existing Conditions," published in May 2010. Estimate 5 is based on the methodology used in the GAO report *Health Insurance: Enrollment, Benefits, Funding, and Other Characteristics of State High-Risk Health Insurance Pools*, GAO-09-730R (Washington, D.C.: July 22, 2009). Information on the conditions included in each estimate is detailed in appendix I. The 95 percent confidence intervals for estimates in this figure are within +/- 1 percent of the estimates themselves.

Figure 2. Percent of Adults (Age 19-64) with Pre-Existing Conditions by Gender, for Low, Midpoint, and High Estimates, 2009.

Compared to individuals with other types of insurance coverage, uninsured adults and those with private individual insurance have the lowest reported rates of pre-existing conditions (see fig. 4). The lower reporting of pre-existing conditions among the uninsured, in part, may reflect the fact that they are less likely than the insured to receive timely preventive care and some common health problems such as hypertension and diabetes often go undetected without routine checkups. In addition, the uninsured are also less likely to have regular preventive care, including cancer screenings.

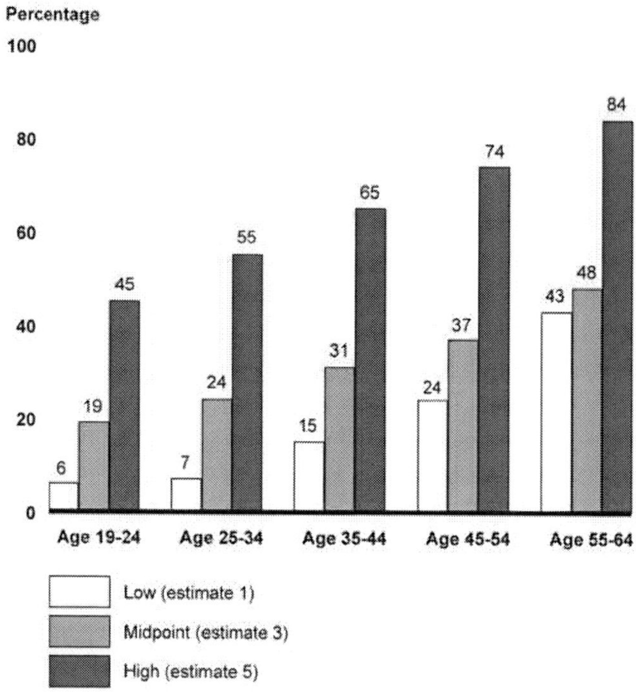

Source: GAO analysis of 2009 Medical Expenditure Panel Survey (MEPS).

Note: Estimate 1 is based on the methodology in Harold Pollack's article "High-Risk Pools for the Sick and Uninsured Under Health Reform: Too Little and Thus Too Late," in the *Journal of General Internal Medicine* (published online on September 2, 2010). Estimate 3 is based on the methodology in the Families USA report "Health Reform: Help for Americans with Pre-Existing Conditions," published in May 2010. Estimate 5 is based on the methodology used in the GAO report *Health Insurance: Enrollment, Benefits, Funding, and Other Characteristics of State High-Risk Health Insurance Pools*, GAO-09-730R (Washington, D.C.: July 22, 2009). Information on the conditions included in each estimate is detailed in appendix I. The 95 percent confidence intervals for estimates in this figure are within +/- 3 percent of the estimates themselves.

Figure 3. Percent of Adults (Age 19-64) with Pre-Existing Conditions within Age Groups for Low, Midpoint, and High Estimates, 2009.

Table 4. Percent of Adults (Age 19-64) with Pre-Existing Conditions within Race and Ethnicity Groups for Low, Midpoint, and High Estimates, 2009

	Low: estimate 1 (percentage)	Midpoint: estimate 3 (percentage)	High: estimate 5 (percentage)
All adults	**20**	**32**	**66**
Asian/Pacific Islander, non-Hispanic	11	15	52
Hispanic	13	26	51
Black, non-Hispanic	19	34	59
White, non-Hispanic	22	35	72
Other, non-Hispanic[a]	[b]	42	67

Source: GAO analysis of Medical Expenditure Panel Survey (MEPS).

Notes: Estimate 1 is based on the methodology in Harold Pollack's article "High-Risk Pools for the Sick and Uninsured Under Health Reform: Too Little and Thus Too Late," in the *Journal of General Internal Medicine* (published online on September 2, 2010). Estimate 3 is based on the methodology in the Families USA report "Health Reform: Help for Americans with Pre-Existing Conditions," published in May 2010. Estimate 5 is based on the methodology used in the GAO report *Health Insurance: Enrollment, Benefits, Funding, and Other Characteristics of State High-Risk Health Insurance Pools*, GAO-09-730R (Washington, D.C.: July 22, 2009). Information on the conditions included in each estimate is detailed in appendix I. The 95 percent confidence intervals for estimates in this table are within +/- 6 percent of the estimates themselves.

[a]Other, non-Hispanic includes American Indians, Alaskan Natives, and individuals identifying with multiple, non-Hispanic races.

[b]Sample size was insufficient to generate a reliable estimate.

The lower reporting of pre-existing conditions among those with private individual insurance may be a reflection of the fact that insurers try to limit the number of people with pre-existing conditions that they accept into their plan.[25] The greatest protections for individuals with pre-existing conditions exist in employer-sponsored group insurance and public insurance programs, which are the groups that reported the highest rates of pre-existing conditions.[26] As noted previously, group insurance plans are not allowed to deny insurance coverage or increase an individual's premiums based on health status. Such protections may encourage individuals in employer group coverage or government insurance to maintain their coverage should they be diagnosed with certain medical conditions. We recently reported that research has consistently found that after a health diagnosis, workers with employer-sponsored coverage were less likely to leave a job or reduce their hours compared to workers who did not rely on their employer for health coverage.[27]

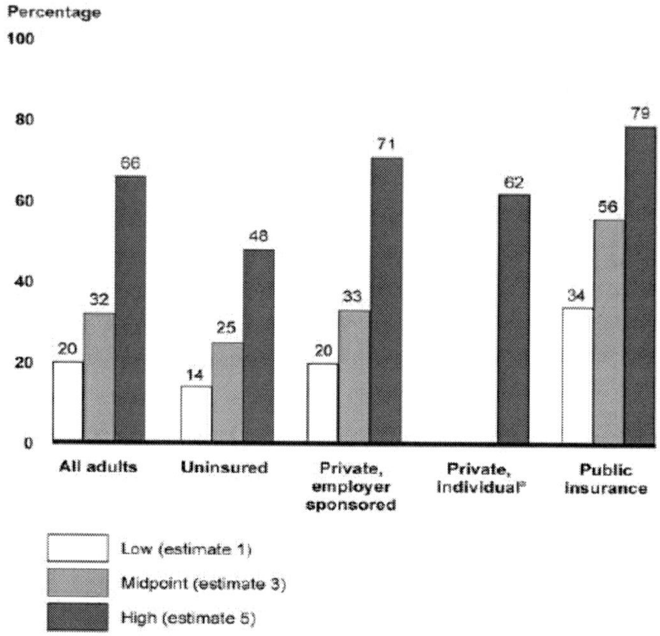

Source: GAO analysis of 2009 Medical Expenditure Panel Survey (MEPS).

Note: Public insurance category includes Medicaid and military health coverage. Estimate 1 is based on the methodology in Harold Pollack's article "High-Risk Pools for the Sick and Uninsured Under Health Reform: Too Little and Thus Too Late," in the *Journal of General Internal Medicine* (published online on September 2, 2010). Estimate 3 is based on the methodology in the Families USA report "Health Reform: Help for Americans with Pre-Existing Conditions," published in May 2010. Estimate 5 is based on the methodology used in the GAO report *Health Insurance: Enrollment, Benefits, Funding, and Other Characteristics of State High-Risk Health Insurance Pools*, GAO-09-730R (Washington, D.C.: July 22, 2009). Estimates are provided only where there was sufficient sample size to generate a reliable estimate. The 95 percent confidence intervals for estimates in this figure are within +/- 7 percent of the estimates themselves.

[a]Only the high estimate for individuals with private, individual insurance had sufficient sample size to generate a reliable estimate.

Figure 4. Percent of Adults (Age 19-64) with Pre-Existing Conditions within Insurance Coverage Groups for Low, Midpoint, and High Estimates, 2009.

Adults with Pre-Existing Conditions Spend Thousands of Dollars More Per Year on Health Care Than Other Adults, but Pre-Existing Conditions Are Common across All Family Income Levels

Adults with pre-existing conditions, on average, spend thousands of dollars more for all health care—between $1,504 and $4,844 more per year—than other adults. Based on the set of conditions included in estimate 1, which included the smallest number of individuals with preexisting conditions, average annual health care expenditures were $8,535 in 2009, compared to $3,691 for all adults (see fig. 5).[28] The average expenditures for the midpoint estimate (estimate 3) were $7,296 and the average expenditures for the high estimate (estimate 5) were $5,195.

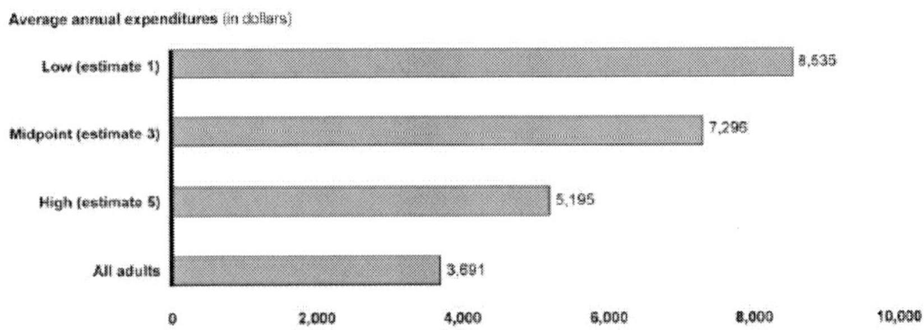

Source: GAO analysis of 2009 Medical Expenditure Panel Survey (MEPS).

Note: Estimate 1 is based on the methodology in Harold Pollack's article "High-Risk Pools for the Sick and Uninsured Under Health Reform: Too Little and Thus Too Late," in the *Journal of General Internal Medicine* (published online on September 2, 2010). Estimate 3 is based on the methodology in the Families USA report "Health Reform: Help for Americans with Pre-Existing Conditions," published in May 2010. Estimate 5 is based on the methodology used in the GAO report *Health Insurance: Enrollment, Benefits, Funding, and Other Characteristics of State High-Risk Health Insurance Pools*, GAO-09-730R (Washington, D.C.: July 22, 2009). Information on the conditions included in each estimate is detailed in appendix I. The 95 percent confidence intervals for estimates in this figure are within +/- 8 percent of the estimates themselves.

Figure 5. Average Annual Health Care Expenditures for Adults (Age 19-64) and among the Low, Midpoint, and High Estimates of Adults with Pre-Existing Conditions, 2009.

Average medical expenditures among those with pre-existing conditions decreased as the number of people in the estimate reporting a preexisting condition increased. As more individuals are included in the estimate, it is likely that the average severity of the medical conditions decreases, thus decreasing the average expenditure estimate. The distribution of adults across income groups, whether measured by total family income or income as a share of the federal poverty level, is similar, regardless of pre-existing condition status (see tables 5 and 6). We found that the average annual family income for adults with preexisting conditions was between $64,000 and $71,000, as compared to the average family income of all adults, which is about $69,000.

Table 5. Distribution of All Adults (Age 19-64) and Those with Pre-Existing Conditions across Total Family Income Categories, Low, Midpoint, and High Estimates, 2009

		Adults with pre-existing conditions (percentage)		
	All adults (percentage)	**Low: estimate 1**	**Midpoint: estimate 3**	**High: estimate 5**
Under $25,000	21	25	25	21
$25,000-$49,999	24	23	24	23
$50,000-$74,999	19	18	18	19
$75,000-$99,999	14	14	14	14
$100,000 and above	22	21	19	23
Total	**100**	**100**	**100**	**100**

Source: GAO analysis of Medical Expenditure Panel Survey (MEPS).

Notes: Income includes annual earnings from wages salaries and other sources including: bonuses, tips, child support payments, Social Security, worker's compensation, veterans' payments, and welfare payments from public assistance and related programs. It does not include tax refunds and capital gains. Estimate 1 is based on the methodology in Harold Pollack's article "High-Risk Pools for the Sick and Uninsured Under Health Reform: Too Little and Thus Too Late," in the *Journal of General Internal Medicine* (published online on September 2, 2010). Estimate 3 is based on the methodology in the Families USA report "Health Reform: Help for Americans with Pre-Existing Conditions," published in May 2010. Estimate 5 is based on the methodology used in the GAO report *Health Insurance: Enrollment, Benefits, Funding, and Other Characteristics of State High-Risk Health Insurance Pools*, GAO-09-730R (Washington, D.C.: July 22, 2009). Total may be greater than 100 percent because of rounding. The 95 percent confidence intervals for estimates in this table are within +/- 2 percent of the estimates themselves.

Table 6. Distribution of All Adults (Age 19-64) and Those with Pre-Existing Conditions across Categories of Family Income as Percent of Poverty Level, Low, Midpoint, and High Estimates, 2009

Income as a percentage of FPL	All Adults (percentage)	Adults with pre-existing conditions (percentage)		
		Low: estimate 1	Midpoint: estimate 3	High: estimate 5
Less than100%	13	15	15	12
100 to 199%	16	16	17	15
200 to 399%	30	28	30	29
Greater than or equal to 400%	41	42	38	44
Total	100	100	100	100

Source: GAO analysis of Medical Expenditure Panel Survey (MEPS).

Notes: Income includes annual earnings from wages salaries and other sources including: bonuses, tips, child support payments, Social Security, worker's compensation, veterans' payments, and welfare payments from public assistance and related programs. It does not include tax refunds and capital gains. Estimate 1 is based on the methodology in Harold Pollack's article "High-Risk Pools for the Sick and Uninsured Under Health Reform: Too Little and Thus Too Late," in the *Journal of General Internal Medicine* (published online on September 2, 2010). Estimate 3 is based on the methodology in the Families USA report "Health Reform: Help for Americans with Pre-Existing Conditions," published in May 2010. Estimate 5 is based on the methodology used in the GAO report *Health Insurance: Enrollment, Benefits, Funding, and Other Characteristics of State High-Risk Health Insurance Pools*, GAO-09-730R (Washington, D.C.: July 22, 2009). Total may be greater than 100 percent because of rounding. The 95 percent confidence intervals for estimates in this table are within +/- 2 percent of the estimates themselves.

AGENCY COMMENTS

We provided a draft of this report to HHS for comment, but in its written response HHS said that it had no substantive or technical comments. HHS noted that PPACA provided individuals with pre-existing conditions new protections, including the opportunity to enroll in the Pre-existing Condition Insurance Plan and the prohibition on insurers limiting or denying insurance coverage because of a pre-existing condition beginning in 2014.

John E. Dicken, Director, Health Care

APPENDIX I: SCOPE AND METHODOLOGY

To answer all of our research objectives, we (1) identified different sets of medical conditions that researchers have used to define the conditions that would cause an insurance company to deny health insurance coverage, offer coverage at higher-than-average premiums, or restrict health insurance coverage; and (2) analyzed data from the 2009 Medical Expenditure Panel Survey (MEPS). We chose the MEPS because it is nationally representative of the civilian, noninstitutionalized population, provides information on medical conditions, medical expenditures, and demographics, and has been used by other researchers to answer similar research objectives.[1] We limited our analysis to adults, defined as individuals age 19 to 64, and we excluded approximately 2.7 million adults continuously enrolled in Medicare in all 12 months of 2009. Based on Medicare eligibility rules, all of these individuals would have a medical condition.

Identifying Pre-Existing Conditions

We identified four previous studies that used different lists of pre-existing conditions to develop five estimates of the number of individuals with pre-existing conditions or the number of individuals potentially eligible for high-risk pools. Because high-risk pools are designed for individuals who cannot obtain insurance in the private individual market because of a preexisting condition, estimates of individuals potentially eligible for high-risk pools can serve as a proxy for individuals with pre-existing conditions. Each of the previous studies looked at different populations, used different years of data, and, in one case, a different source of data. We assigned each condition list an estimate number from 1 to 5 in order to more readily identify which set of conditions was associated with each estimate.[2] For example, the condition list in the study authored by Harold Pollack is referred to as estimate 1.

Estimate 1 is based on the condition list in Harold Pollack's article "High-Risk Pools for the Sick and Uninsured Under Health Reform: Too Little and Thus Too Late," in the *Journal of General Internal Medicine* (published online on September 2, 2010). Pollack considered individuals to be plausible high-risk pool participants if they had ever been told they had emphysema, diabetes, stroke, cancer, congestive heart failure, heart disease, angina, or heart attack.

Estimate 2 is described below with the information on estimate 4 because both estimates came from the same study. Additionally, estimate 2 is based on the methodology used in estimate 3.

Estimate 3 is based on the condition list in the Families USA report "Health Reform: Help for Americans with Pre-Existing Conditions," published in May 2010. According to a methodology developed by researchers from The Lewin Group, individuals were identified as having a pre-existing condition if they reported, in the previous year, one of 67 conditions most commonly included in lists for determining high-risk pool eligibility across all the states with high-risk pools. The conditions were: acquired immune deficiency syndrome (AIDS), alcohol/drug abuse/chemical dependency, Alzheimer's disease, angina pectoris, anorexia nervosa, aplastic anemia, aortic aneurysm, arteriosclerosis obliterans, artificial heart valve/heart valve replacement, ascites, brain tumor, cancer (except skin), cancer (metastatic), cardiomyopathy/primary cardiomyopathy, cerebral palsy/palsy, chronic obstructive pulmonary disease (COPD), chronic pancreatitis, cirrhosis of the liver, congestive heart failure, coronary artery disease, coronary insufficiency, coronary occlusion, Crohn's disease, cystic fibrosis, dermatomyositis, diabetes, emphysema/pulmonary emphysema, Friedreich's disease/ataxia, hemophilia, hepatitis, HIV positive, Hodgkin's disease, Huntington's chorea/disease, hydrocephalus, intermittent claudication, kidney failure/kidney disease with dialysis/renal failure, lead poisoning with cerebral involvement, leukemia, Lou Gehrig's disease/amytrophic lateral sclerosis/ALS, lupus erythematosus disseminate/lupus, major organ transplant, malignant tumor, mood and psychotic disorders (including depression, schizophrenia, and bipolar disorder), motor or sensory aphasia, multiple or disseminated sclerosis, muscular atrophy or dystrophy, myasthenia gravis, myocardial infarction (heart attack), myotonia, obesity, paraplegia or quadriplegia, Parkinson's disease, peripheral arteriosclerosis, polyarteritis, polycystic kidney, postero-lateral sclerosis, rheumatoid arthritis, sickle cell anemia/sickle cell disease, silicosis, splenic anemia/True Banti's Syndrome/Banti's disease, Still's disease, stroke, syringomyelia (spina bifida or myelomeningocele), tabes dorsalis, thalassemia (Cooley's or Mediterranean anemia), ulcerative colitis, and Wilson's disease.

Estimates 2 and 4 were based on the two condition lists in the Department of Health and Human Services' (HHS) report "At Risk: Pre-Existing Conditions Could Affect 1 in 2 Americans: 129 Million People Could Be Denied Affordable Coverage Without Health Reform" (Washington, D.C.: January 2011). This report included two estimates of individuals with pre-existing conditions. Estimate 2 replicated the methodology developed by The Lewin Group for the Families USA study with two exceptions. First, obesity was not included in the list of conditions that would cause a denial because HHS researchers did not find obesity on the condition lists used by state high-risk pools. Second, HHS included individuals who reported that they had ever been diagnosed with the following conditions: coronary heart disease, myocardial infarction, other heart disease, angina pectoris, stroke, emphysema, cancer, and diabetes. HHS's second estimate, estimate 4, included the same conditions as its first estimate with additional conditions added based on a review of the underwriting guidelines of seven health insurers. In addition to the conditions included in estimate 2, estimate 4 included individuals reporting arthritis, asthma, high cholesterol, hypertension, or obesity, as well as those who had ever been diagnosed with arthritis, asthma, high cholesterol, or hypertension. Estimate 4 also includes individuals reporting neurotic and related disorders, stress and adjustment disorders, conduct disorders, and emotional disturbances.

Estimate 5 was based on the methodology used in the GAO report *Health Insurance: Enrollment, Benefits, Funding, and Other Characteristics of State High-Risk Health Insurance Pools*, GAO-09-730R (Washington, D.C.: July 22, 2009). This report used the Healthcare Cost and Utilization Project's Chronic Condition Indicator to identify chronic conditions in the 2006 MEPS, which were assumed to make a person medically uninsurable and therefore potentially eligible for a state high-risk pool. The Chronic Condition Indicator categorizes all International Classification of Diseases, Ninth Edition, Clinical Modification (ICD-9-CM) codes as chronic or not chronic.[3] A chronic condition is defined as a condition that lasts 12 months or longer and meets one or both of the following tests: (a) it places limitations on self-care, independent living, and social interactions; and (b) it results in the need for ongoing intervention with medical products, services, and special equipment. Individuals reporting any condition considered chronic were included in this estimate. We used the three-digit ICD-9-CM codes for medical conditions. Of 1,019 three-digit ICD-9-CM codes, the Chronic Condition Indicator categorized 417 as chronic.

To standardize the estimates from the different sources, we applied the conditions identified by each study to the same population (19 to 64 year olds not enrolled in Medicare) and the same year and source of data (the 2009 MEPS) to construct estimates 1 through 5.

Identifying the Most Common Medical Conditions and Estimating Treatment Costs

To estimate the number of adults (age 19 to 64) with medical conditions that would cause an insurance company to restrict or deny insurance coverage and the average expenditures related to these conditions, we analyzed MEPS data on medical conditions and expenditures. We reported data only for those medical conditions included in at least one of the condition lists used for estimates 1 through 5. MEPS respondents report medical conditions identified as the reason for a medical event, the reason for a disability day, or as something that is "bothering" the respondent during the reference year (in this case, 2009).[4] To protect respondent privacy, we only reported estimates based on sample sizes of 100 or more. We defined expenditures as payments from all sources for hospital inpatient care, ambulatory care provided in offices and hospital outpatient departments, care provided in emergency departments, and the purchase of prescribed medications.[5] We did not include expenditures for dental expenses or other medical expenses, such as durable and nondurable supplies, medical equipment, eyeglasses, and ambulance services because these items could not be linked to specific conditions. We also excluded expenses for home health care. We classified expenditures with a condition if a visit, stay, or medication purchase was cited as being related to the specific condition.

Demographic and Geographic Profile of Adults with Pre-Existing Conditions

To describe the demographic and geographic profile of adults with pre-existing conditions we focused on the low, midpoint, and high estimates of adults with pre-existing conditions, which we call estimates 1, 3, and 5, respectively. We provided state estimates for the 35 states with sufficient sample size in the MEPS data to reliably report an estimate. We did not have large enough sample sizes to generate state-level estimates of the number of adults with pre-existing conditions in Alaska, Delaware, Idaho, Maine, Montana, Nebraska, Nevada, New Hampshire, New Mexico, North Dakota, Rhode Island, South Dakota, Vermont, West Virginia, Wyoming, and the District of Columbia. To estimate the number of individuals living in states with insurance protections similar to those that will be offered under PPACA in 2014, we surveyed state insurance department officials in September 2011, asking them to confirm or correct information on guaranteed issue requirements and rating restrictions previously reported by the Kaiser Family Foundation's statehealthfacts.org website.[6] We asked the state officials to confirm information on guaranteed issue requirements and rating restrictions in place as of September 2011. We received responses from all states and the District of Columbia. Based on those responses, we used MEPS's state-based estimates of adults age 19 to 64 with preexisting conditions to identify the number of individuals living in states reporting a guaranteed issue requirement for at least some policies and either pure community rating or adjusted community rating—insurance protections similar to those that will be offered under PPACA in 2014. Guaranteed issue requirements prohibit the denial of coverage to individuals based on pre-existing conditions. In some states, all products must be guaranteed issue, while in other states guaranteed issue requirements are only applicable to some individuals, for instance those with 12 months of continuous coverage, or some standard product, such as a basic health plan. Under pure community rating, insurers may not adjust premiums based on health status, age, or gender. Under adjusted community rating, insurers may not adjust premiums based on health status, but may adjust premiums based on characteristics such as gender or age, depending on the state.

Study Limitations and Data Reliability

There are limitations to our analysis. First, each insurance company separately determines which medical conditions will result in a denial, limitation in coverage, or an increase in premiums. An individual who may be denied by one insurer could obtain coverage from another. Therefore, the population of individuals who would be denied by an insurer, offered restricted coverage, or offered coverage at higher-than-average premiums actually varies by each health insurer. Second, our estimates could overstate the adult population with pre-existing conditions because of the way in which conditions are aggregated in the MEPS database. To protect survey participant confidentiality, five-digit ICD-9-CM codes are truncated into a three-digit code, which means that individuals reporting other related conditions may also be captured. To determine the reliability of the MEPS data, we reviewed related documentation, compared our estimates to other published results, and spoke with an official from the Agency for Healthcare Research and Quality, which is the federal agency responsible for MEPS. We determined that the

MEPS data were sufficiently reliable for the purposes of our engagement. The 2009 data are the most recently available for MEPS. We conducted this performance audit in accordance with generally accepted government auditing standards from July 2011 through March 2012. Those standards require that we plan and perform the audit to obtain sufficient, appropriate evidence to provide a reasonable basis for our findings and conclusions based on our audit objectives. We believe that the evidence obtained provides a reasonable basis for our findings based on our audit objectives.

APPENDIX II: NUMBER OF ADULTS (AGE 19-64) WITH PRE-EXISTING CONDITIONS IN STATES, LOW, MIDPOINT, AND HIGH ESTIMATE, 2009

State	Low: estimate 1		Midpoint: estimate 3		High: estimate 5	
	Number	Standard error	Number	Standard error	Number	Standard error
All adults	36,116,647	1,056,380	59,978,301	1,734,242	121,560,174	2,950,667
Alabama	—	—	—	—	1,936,170[a]	692,379
Alaska	—	—	—	—	—	—
Arizona	—	—	1,136,752	304,102	2,216,186	501,837
Arkansas	—	—	—	—	1,480,153[a]	755,180
California	4,004,774	511,259	6,606,715	857,916	13,651,336	1,435,726
Colorado	—	—	—	—	1,893,776[a]	590,540
Connecticut	—	—	—	—	1,211,605[a]	618,166
Delaware	—	—	—	—	—	—
District of Columbia	—	—	—	—	—	—
Florida	1,670,935	255,058	2,612,694	384,664	5,689,120	906,300
Georgia	1,215,469	136,640	1,898,146	211,029	3,461,859	301,183
Hawaii	—	—	—	—	683,798[a]	348,877
Idaho	—	—	—	—	—	—
Illinois	1,179,171	159,490	2,181,909	343,397	4,488,169	575,415
Indiana	—	—	1,358,572	233,200	2,623,593	408,833
Iowa	—	—	—	—	1,597,729	349,209
Kansas	—	—	—	—	1,047,433[a]	534,405
Kentucky	—	—	2,186,644[a]	1,058,849	3,527,324[a]	1,699,657
Louisiana	—	—	—	—	1,436,715[a]	590,999
Maine	—	—	—	—	—	—
Maryland	—	—	—	—	2,161,840	370,581
Massachusetts	—	—	1,097,055	271,483	2,311,677	550,103
Michigan	1,226,779	221,142	2,453,149	495,322	4,390,757	888,570
Minnesota	—	—	—	—	2,333,096	347,476
Mississippi	—	—	—	—	1,432,693[a]	730,966

(Continued)

State	Low: estimate 1		Midpoint: estimate 3		High: estimate 5	
	Number	Standard error	Number	Standard error	Number	Standard error
Missouri	—	—	1,407,053	210,782	2,736,950	444,142
Montana	—	—	—	—	—	—
Nebraska	—	—	—	—	—	—
Nevada	—	—	—	—	—	—
New Hampshire	—	—	—	—	—	—
New Jersey	1,055,825	142,155	1,914,939	293,777	4,474,967	690,321
New Mexico	—	—	—	—	—	—
New York	1,952,701	524,780	3,580,631	876,213	7,308,236	1,725,171
North Carolina	1,131,189[a]	553,188	1,746,407[a]	891,024	3,426,132[a]	1,748,027
North Dakota	—	—	—	—	—	—
Ohio	1,758,412	358,372	2,523,454	540,527	4,945,135	837,152
Oklahoma	—	—	—	—	1,230,321[a]	627,715
Oregon	—	—	—	—	2,008,453[a]	867,185
Pennsylvania	1,628,060	139,301	2,777,003	271,756	5,546,111	583,727
Rhode Island	—	—	—	—	—	—
South Carolina	—	—	—	—	1,324,442[a]	675,736
South Dakota	—	—	—	—	—	—
Tennessee	—	—	772,781[a]	394,276	1,625,348[a]	829,259
Texas	2,673,379	378,510	4,366,855	619,441	9,045,432	1,483,132
Utah	—	—	—	—	1,736,201[a]	885,817
Vermont	—	—	—	—	—	—
Virginia	1,160,804[a]	380,094	1,895,256	541,223	3,968,986	1,137,964
Washington	—	—	1,509,783	328,015	3,542,050	736,548
West Virginia	—	—	—	—	—	—
Wisconsin	—	—	—	—	2,319,211[a]	834,253
Wyoming	—	—	—	—	—	—

Source: GAO analysis of Medical Expenditure Panel Survey (MEPS).

Notes: Information on the conditions included in each estimate is detailed in appendix I. Estimate 1 is based on the methodology in Harold Pollack's article "High-Risk Pools for the Sick and Uninsured Under Health Reform: Too Little and Thus Too Late," in the *Journal of General Internal Medicine* (published online on September 2, 2010). Estimate 3 is based on the methodology in the Families USA report "Health Reform: Help for Americans with Pre-Existing Conditions," published in May 2010. Estimate 5 is based on the methodology used in the GAO report *Health Insurance: Enrollment, Benefits, Funding, and Other Characteristics of State High-Risk Health Insurance Pools*, GAO-09-730R (Washington, D.C.: July 22, 2009). The standard error is a measure of variation around the estimate, in this case, the estimated number of individuals in the state with pre-existing conditions. The 95 percent confidence intervals for estimates in this table are within +/- 3 percent of the estimates themselves. Due to insufficient sample sizes, MEPS data could not be used to provide any estimates for 15 states and Washington, D.C. Dashes in the table indicate that the sample size was not sufficient to produce an estimate.

[a]The relative standard error is greater than or equal to 30 percent. Relative standard error is the proportion of the standard error divided by the estimate itself.

APPENDIX III: STATE PROTECTIONS FOR INDIVIDUALS WITH PRE-EXISTING CONDITIONS, AS OF SEPTEMBER 2011

State	Guaranteed issue[a]	Insurer of last resort[b]	Pure community rating[c]	Adjusted community rating[d]	Rate bands[e]
Alabama	No	No	No	No	No
Alaska	No	No	No	No	No
Arizona	Yes - Some	No	No	No	No
Arkansas	No	No	No	No	No
California	No	No	No	No	No
Colorado	No	No	No	No	No
Connecticut	No	No	No	No	No
Delaware	No	No	No	No	No
District of Columbia	No	No	No	No	No
Florida	No	No	No	No	No
Georgia	No	No	No	No	No
Hawaii	No	No	No	No	No
Idaho	Yes - Some	No	No	No	Yes
Illinois	No	No	No	No	No
Indiana	No	No	No	No	No
Iowa	No	No	No	No	Yes
Kansas	No	No	No	No	No
Kentucky	No	No	No	No	Yes
Louisiana	No	No	No	f No	Yes
Maine	Yes - All	No	No	Yes	No
Maryland	No	No	No	No	Yes
Massachusetts	Yes – All	No	No	Yes	No
Michigan	Yes – Some	No	No	No	No
Minnesota	No	No	No	No	Yes
Mississippi	No	No	No	No	No
Missouri	No	No	No	No	No
Montana	No	No	No	No	No
Nebraska	No	No	No	No	No
Nevada	No	No	No	No	Yes
New Hampshire	No	No	No	No	Yes
New Jersey	Yes – All	No[g]	No	Yes	No
New Mexico	No	No	No	No	Yes
New York	Yes – All	No	Yes	No	No
North Carolina	No	No	No	No	No
North Dakota	No	No	No	No	No
Ohio	Yes – Some	No	No	No	No[h]
Oklahoma	No	No	No	No	No
Oregon	No	No	No	Yes	No

(Continued)

State	Guaranteed issuea	Insurer of last resortb	Pure community ratingc	Adjusted community ratingd	Rate bandse
Pennsylvania	No	Yes	No	Yes	No
Rhode Island	Yes – Some	Yes	No	No	No
South Carolina	No	No	No	No	No
South Dakota	No	No	No	No	Yes
Tennessee	No	No	No	No	Yes
Texas	No	No	No	No	No
Utah	Yes – Some	No	No	No	Yes
Vermont	Yes – All	No	No	Yes	No
Virginia	No	Yes	No	No	No
Washington	No	No	No	Yes	No
West Virginia	Yes – Some	No	No	No	No
Wisconsin	No	No	No	No	No
Wyoming	No	No	No	No	No

Source: GAO survey of state officials pertaining to categories of protection previously reported on by the Kaiser Family Foundation.

Note: We did not attempt to independently identify categories of protection or to validate the accuracy of the state responses.

[a]Guaranteed issue requirements prohibit the denial of coverage to individuals based on pre-existing conditions. In some states, all products must be guaranteed issue, while in other states guaranteed issue requirements are only applicable to some individuals, for instance those with 12 months of creditable coverage, or some standard product, such as a basic health plan.

[b]An insurer of last resort law requires one insurer in the state to issue products to individuals regardless of pre-existing conditions.

[c]Under pure community rating, insurers may not adjust premiums due to health status, age, or gender.

[d]Under adjusted community rating, insurers may not adjust premiums due to health status, but may adjust premiums according to characteristics such as gender or age, depending on the state.

[e]Rate bands limit the extent to which premium can vary based on an individual's health status, for example, to a certain percentage of the average premium.

[f]Louisiana reported that its community modified rating law allows for limited rate variation between member participants for health status, tier rating, and durational rating. It also allows rating for age, gender, industry, geographic area, family composition, group size, tobacco usage, plan of benefits, or other factors approved by the Louisiana Department of Insurance.

[g]While New Jersey reported that it has an insurer of last resort by law, it does not function as such in practice because of the guaranteed issue requirement.

[h]Rating bands only apply in parts of the individual market where a small group plan is being converted to an individual plan.

End Notes

[1] Medicare is a federal health care program that provides health insurance for those aged 65 and older, certain disabled persons, and persons with end-stage renal disease. Medicaid is a joint federal-state program that finances health care coverage for certain low-income individuals.

[2]Percentages do not sum to 100 because estimates of coverage types are not mutually exclusive and individuals can have more than one type of coverage during the year. Data from the Census Bureau on adults is available for 18-64 year olds. See C. DeNavas-Walt, B.D. Proctor, and J.C. Smith, U.S. Census Bureau, *Current Population Reports, P60-239, Income, Poverty, and Health Insurance Coverage in the United States: 2010* (Washington, D.C.: 2011).

[3] Individuals not eligible to purchase employer-sponsored group coverage may buy coverage in the private individual market; these include the self-employed; those whose employers do not offer health insurance coverage; individuals not in the labor force; early retirees who no longer have employment-based coverage and are not yet eligible for Medicare; and individuals who lose their jobs and are either ineligible for or have exhausted the right to continue their employer-based coverage for 18 months.

[4] Pub. L. No. 111-148, 124 Stat. 119 (Mar. 23, 2010), as amended by the Health Care and Education Reconciliation Act of 2010 (HCERA), Pub. L. No. 111-152, 124 Stat. 1029 (Mar. 30, 2010). For purposes of this report, references to PPACA include the amendments made by HCERA.

[5] Pub. L. No. 111-148, § 1201, 124 Stat. 154 (adding § 2704 to the Public Health Service Act (PHSA)). Although a PPACA provision prohibiting denials of coverage or restrictions on benefits because of a pre-existing condition for individuals under the age of 19 became effective September 23, 2010, insurers can still vary premium rates based on health status for these individuals until 2014. *See* Pub. L. No. 111-148 § 11253 as amended by § 10103(e), 124 Stat. 162, 895.

[6] A panel survey involves multiple interviews with respondents over time.

[7] During interviews, household respondents are asked about medical events, and after completing the interview (and obtaining permission), researchers contact a sample of medical providers by telephone to obtain information that the respondents may not be able to provide accurately, such as visit dates, diagnosis and procedure codes, charges, and payments.

[8] High-risk pools are designed for individuals who cannot obtain insurance in the individual market because of a pre-existing condition, and therefore estimates of individuals potentially eligible for high-risk pools can serve as a proxy for individuals with pre-existing conditions.

[9] A chronic condition is defined as one that lasts 12 months or longer and places limits on self-care, independent living, and social interactions and/or results in the need for ongoing intervention.

[10] See GAO, *Private Health Insurance: Data on Application and Coverage Denials*, GAO-11-268 (Washington, D.C.: Mar. 16, 2011). The information is based on data collected by Department of Health and Human Services (HHS).

[11] America's Health Insurance Plans' Center for Policy and Research, *Individual Health Insurance 2009: A Comprehensive Survey of Premiums, Availability, and Benefits* (Washington, D.C.: October 2009). America's Health Insurance Plans is the national trade association representing the health insurance industry. According to the study, 84 percent of applications were medically underwritten. Just over 1 percent of applications were denied

before going through medical underwriting, but those denials were unrelated to the applicant's health status.

[12] *See* Pub. L. No. 104-191, Title I, 110 Stat. 1936, 1939 et. seq.

[13] Pub. L. No.104-191, § 111, 110 Stat. 1978 (adding 2741 to the PHSA). Creditable coverage is defined for this purpose by §2701(c)(1) of the PHSA as coverage for an individual under: a group health plan, health insurance, Medicare Part A or B, Medicaid, TRICARE, the Indian Health Service or a tribal organization, a state health benefits high-risk pool, the Federal Employees Health Benefits Program, the Peace Corps health benefit plan, or a public health plan as defined in regulations.

[14] Thirty-five states have state high-risk pools: Alabama, Alaska, Arkansas, California, Colorado, Connecticut, Florida, Idaho, Indiana, Illinois, Iowa, Kansas, Kentucky, Louisiana, Maryland, Minnesota, Mississippi, Missouri, Montana, Nebraska, New Hampshire, New Mexico, North Carolina, North Dakota, Oklahoma, Oregon, South Carolina, South Dakota, Tennessee, Texas, Utah, Washington, West Virginia, Wisconsin, and Wyoming.

[15] Pub. L. No. 111-148, § 1101, 124 Stat. 141.

[16] See GAO, *Pre-Existing Condition Insurance Plans: Program Features, Early Enrollment and Spending Trends, and Federal Oversight Activities*, GAO-11-662 (Washington, D.C.: July 27, 2011).

[17] Estimates are of individuals who reported that these conditions were the cause of a medical event, the reason for a disability day, or bothered a respondent during 2009.

[18] Expenditure information is reported only for those with expenditures greater than $0 and includes expenditures from all sources for hospital inpatient stays, emergency room visits, outpatient department visits, office-based medical provider visits, and prescribed medicines. Expenditure information does not include amounts for dental expenses and other medical expenses, such as durable and nondurable supplies, medical equipment, eyeglasses, and ambulance services because these items could not be linked to specific conditions. We also did not include expenditures for home health care.

[19] Mental health disorders are defined as mood and psychotic disorders, which include conditions such as depression, bipolar disorder, and schizophrenia.

[20] The eight conditions are: angina pectoris, cancer, congestive heart failure, diabetes, emphysema, heart attack (myocardial infarction), other heart disease, and stroke.

[21] A chronic condition is defined as a condition that lasts 12 months or longer and meets one or both of the following tests: (a) it places limitations on self-care, independent living, and social interactions; and (b) it results in the need for ongoing intervention with medical products, services, and special equipment. Examples of chronic conditions include malignancies, diabetes, most forms of mental illness, hypertension, many forms of heart disease, and congenital anomalies. Nonchronic conditions include conditions such as infections, pregnancy, many neonatal conditions, nonspecific symptoms, and injuries. We determined which conditions were considered chronic by using the Healthcare Cost and Utilization Project's Chronic Care Indicator, which categorizes medical conditions as either chronic or nonchronic conditions. Out of a total of 1,019 3-digit International Classification of Diseases, Ninth Edition, Clinical Modification (ICD-9-CM) codes, we identified 417 as chronic conditions. ICD-9-CM is a commonly used system to classify and code medical conditions.

[22] Due to insufficient sample sizes, MEPS data could not be used to provide estimates for 15 states and the District of Columbia. The 15 states are Alaska, Delaware, Idaho, Maine, Montana, North Dakota, Nebraska, New Hampshire, New Mexico, Nevada, Rhode Island, South Dakota, Vermont, Wyoming, and West Virginia.

[23] Guaranteed issue, pure community rating, and adjusted community rating are defined on pages 6-7.

[24] Pregnancy was not considered a pre-existing condition in any of the studies we reviewed.

[25] Due to insufficient sample sizes, we were only able to generate an estimate of individuals in the private individual market reporting pre-existing conditions for the high estimate (estimate 5).

[26] Public insurance programs include Medicaid and military health coverage. For the purposes of our report, we excluded individuals with Medicare from our analysis.

[27] GAO, *Health Care Coverage: Job Lock and the Potential Impact of the Patient Protection and Affordable Care Act*, GAO-12-166R (Washington, D.C.: Dec. 15, 2011).

[28] Annual expenditures on health care included expenditures on any medical condition during the year. Individuals with pre-existing conditions can have multiple medical conditions.

End Notes for Appendix I

[1] During interviews, household respondents are asked about medical events, and after completing the interview (and obtaining permission), researchers contact a sample of medical providers by telephone to obtain information that the respondents may not be able to provide accurately, such as visit dates, diagnosis and procedure codes, charges, and payments.

[2] One study made both a low and high estimate.

[3] ICD-9-CM is a commonly used system to classify and code medical conditions. The Chronic Condition Indicator is one in a family of databases and software tools developed as part of the Healthcare Cost and Utilization Project, a federal-state-industry partnership sponsored by the Agency for Healthcare Research and Quality.

[4] For MEPS, medical conditions were recorded by an interviewer as verbatim text, which was then coded by professional coders to five-digit International Statistical Classification of Diseases, Ninth Revision codes (ICD-9). ICD-9 codes are a commonly used set of codes used to classify medical conditions. The five-digit ICD-9 codes were then aggregated into clinically meaningful categories that group similar conditions, known as Clinical Classification codes. In addition, MEPS includes the ICD-9 code, but truncates it to three-digits to protect the confidentiality of survey participants. When possible, we used the Clinical Classification codes in our analysis. When a medical condition did not align with the conditions noted with the Clinical Classification codes, we used the three-digit ICD-9 code to identify individuals with the condition.

[5] Sources of payment include direct payments from individuals, private insurance, Medicare, Medicaid, Workers' Compensation, and miscellaneous other sources. Payments for over-the-counter drugs are not included in MEPS total expenditures. Indirect payments not related to specific medical events are also excluded.

[6] The Kaiser Family Foundation indicated that the information on this website was collected by the Center for Health Insurance Studies, Georgetown University Health Policy Institute and was current as of January 2011.

In: Health Care in the United States
Editor: Leone Giangiulio
ISBN: 978-1-62618-413-8

Chapter 3

PRIVATE HEALTH INSURANCE: EXPIRATION OF THE HEALTH COVERAGE TAX CREDIT WILL AFFECT PARTICIPANTS' COSTS AND COVERAGE CHOICES AS HEALTH REFORM PROVISIONS ARE IMPLEMENTED*

United States Government Accountability Office

WHY GAO DID THIS STUDY

The HCTC pays 72.5 percent of health plan premiums for certain workers who lost their jobs due to foreign import competition and for certain retirees whose pensions from their former employers were terminated and are now paid by the Pension Benefit Guaranty Corporation. A small share of individuals who are potentially eligible for the HCTC participate. In 2010 there were 43,864 participants and 469,168 nonparticipants. The HCTC program will expire at the end of 2013 when premium tax credits and cost-sharing subsidies become available to eligible individuals who purchase health plans through health insurance exchanges under PPACA. PPACA also

* This is an edited, reformatted and augmented version of United States Government Accountability Office, Publication No. GAO-13-147, dated December 2012.

expands Medicaid eligibility to nonelderly individuals who meet specific income requirements to the extent that states choose to implement this provision. Therefore, the costs for health plans and coverage available to individuals potentially eligible for the HCTC will change when the HCTC expires.

This report examines (1) how the HCTC's expiration and the implementation of the PPACA premium tax credit, cost-sharing subsidies, and Medicaid expansion will affect HCTC participants and nonparticipants, and (2) how the coverage that will be available through the PPACA exchanges compares to HCTC participants' health plan coverage. GAO analyzed 2010 HCTC program data and individual tax filer data. GAO also compared the services and actuarial values of the plans that will be available through the exchanges to HCTC plans.

What GAO Found

Expiration of the Health Coverage Tax Credit (HCTC) and implementation of Patient Protection and Affordable Care Act (PPACA) premium tax credits, cost-sharing subsidies, and Medicaid expansion will affect HCTC participants' costs for health plans in multiple ways. Projections from GAO's analysis of 2010 Internal Revenue Service (IRS) data show that most HCTC participants in 2014 will likely be eligible for less generous tax credits under PPACA than the HCTC. Specifically, about 69 percent of HCTC participants will likely be ineligible for either a PPACA premium tax credit or Medicaid, or they will likely receive a PPACA premium tax credit less generous than the HCTC. On the other hand, GAO's analysis also found that at least 23 percent will likely be eligible for PPACA premium tax credits more generous than the HCTC. In addition to the PPACA premium tax credit, up to 28 percent of all HCTC participants will likely be eligible for PPACA cost-sharing subsidies—subsidies that will help them pay for deductibles and copays—depending in part on whether or not their state expands Medicaid under PPACA. For HCTC nonparticipants, the projections from GAO's analysis of 2010 IRS data show that as many as 30 percent may be eligible for either Medicaid or a PPACA premium tax credit more generous than the HCTC in 2014, depending in part on whether or not their state expands Medicaid and whether they meet all other eligibility criteria for the PPACA premium tax credits.

In general, the health plan coverage that will be available through the PPACA exchanges will be comparable to coverage in HCTC participants' current plans; however, HCTC participants may have an incentive to choose plans through the exchanges that have different levels of coverage than their HCTC plans. Plans purchased through the PPACA exchanges will be required to provide essential health benefits—including coverage for specific service categories, such as ambulatory care, prescription drugs, and hospitalization—and most HCTC plans cover these categories of services. In addition, the vast majority of HCTC plans in 2012 likely had actuarial values—the expected percentage of costs that a plan will incur for services provided to a standard population—above the minimum actuarial value of 60 percent that health plans sold through the PPACA exchanges will be required to meet. However, because the PPACA premium tax credit amount will be based on a plan with an actuarial value of 70 percent, HCTC participants who currently have plans with either higher or lower actuarial values and are eligible for PPACA premium tax credits may have an incentive to choose plans that will have different levels of coverage than their HCTC plans. For example, those who have HCTC plans with actuarial values that are higher than 70 percent may have an incentive to shift to health plans with an actuarial value of 70 percent to avoid paying any difference in premiums that could result from choosing plans with higher actuarial values. Similarly, those who now have plans with actuarial values below 70 percent could have the opposite incentive and may purchase plans that offer a higher level of coverage than their current HCTC plans.

We provided draft copies of this report to the Department of Health and Human Services and IRS for review, and both provided technical comments, which we incorporated as appropriate.

ABBREVIATIONS

CCIIO	Center for Consumer Information and Insurance Oversight
COBRA	Consolidated Omnibus Budget Reconciliation Act
EHB	essential health benefits
FPL	federal poverty level
HCTC	Health Coverage Tax Credit
HHS	Department of Health and Human Services
IRS	Internal Revenue Service
PBGC	Pension Benefit Guaranty Corporation

PPACA	Patient Protection and Affordable Care Act
RTAA	Reemployment Trade Adjustment Assistance
TAA	Trade Adjustment Assistance
VEBA	Voluntary Employees' Beneficiary Association

December 28, 2012
The Honorable Max Baucus
Chairman
Committee on Finance United States Senate

The Honorable John D. Rockefeller, IV
Chairman
Subcommittee on Health Care
Committee on Finance United States Senate

The health coverage tax credit (HCTC) pays a share of health plan premiums for certain workers who lost their jobs because of foreign import competition and who are eligible for benefits in the Trade Adjustment Assistance (TAA) program and for certain retirees age 55 and over whose pensions from a former employer were terminated and are now paid by the Pension Benefit Guaranty Corporation (PBGC). The Trade Adjustment Assistance Reform Act of 2002 established the HCTC, which is administered by the Internal Revenue Service (IRS).[1] The Trade Adjustment Assistance Extension Act of 2011 increased the HCTC from 65 percent to 72.5 percent of health plan premiums and also specified that the HCTC program will expire at the end of 2013.[2] Beginning January 1, 2014, premium tax credits and cost-sharing subsidies— subsidies that will help individuals pay for out-of-pocket expenses such as deductibles and copays—will become available under the Patient Protection and Affordable Care Act (PPACA).[3] These tax credits and subsidies will help eligible individuals pay for the premiums and cost-sharing for health plans purchased through health insurance exchanges created under PPACA.[4] Effective January 1, 2014, PPACA also expands eligibility for Medicaid to nonelderly individuals who meet specific income requirements to the extent that states choose to implement this provision.[5] As a result, individuals who participate in or were potentially eligible for the HCTC may be eligible for Medicaid when the HCTC expires. The IRS will administer the PPACA premium tax credits and the Department of Health and Human Services' (HHS) Center for Consumer Information and Insurance Oversight (CCIIO) will oversee the PPACA exchanges and cost-sharing subsidies.

Although the HCTC pays a significant share of health plan premiums for eligible individuals who participate in the program, participation in the HCTC has been lower than expected. For example, in 2010 less than 10 percent of over 500,000 potentially eligible individuals were participating in the HCTC. In our prior work, we analyzed data from IRS surveys conducted in 2009 of individuals who were potentially eligible for the HCTC. 6 We found that survey respondents most commonly reported improved affordability of health plans as a reason for participation in the HCTC and most commonly reported ineligibility as a reason for not participating.[7] The second most commonly reported reason for not participating was lack of affordability—such as being unable to afford to pay for health plan premiums even with the credit. While HCTC nonparticipants do not currently benefit from the HCTC, some may benefit from PPACA. That is, some may have new incentives to obtain health coverage under PPACA rules, for example if they are eligible for the PPACA premium tax credit, and particularly if they are eligible for a credit that is more generous than the HCTC. In addition, some nonparticipants may be eligible for PPACA cost-sharing subsidies or become newly eligible for Medicaid.

To receive the HCTC, recipients must be enrolled in HCTC-qualified health plans. [8] These include certain group health plans, such as plans that are a continuation of employer-sponsored health plans through the Consolidated Omnibus Budget Reconciliation Act (COBRA)—referred to as COBRA plans throughout this report—and Voluntary Employees' Beneficiary Association (VEBA) plans.[9] The HCTC-qualified health plans also include individual (nongroup) market plans and HCTC state-qualified plans, which can vary in design, but which must ensure certain consumer protections. Similarly, to receive PPACA premium tax credits and cost-sharing subsidies when they become available in 2014, recipients must be enrolled in health plans that are purchased through the PPACA exchanges. These plans will need to meet certain coverage requirements. Specifically, they will be required to provide essential health benefits (EHB) which include coverage for specific service categories, such as hospitalization, prescription drugs, and emergency services.[10] A plan will be identified in each state that specifies what the EHB are for that state— this plan will be referred to as that state's benchmark plan. In addition, plans sold through the PPACA exchanges will be offered at four different levels of coverage corresponding to a percentage of the full actuarial value of plan benefits for EHB and designated by a different metal tier: 60 percent (bronze), 70 percent (silver), 80 percent (gold), and 90 percent (platinum).[11] For the purposes of this report, the term "coverage" includes two elements: (1) the categories of services a plan covers; and (2) a plan's actuarial value, which we refer to as a plan's level of coverage.

Because the HCTC will expire when the PPACA premium tax credit and cost-sharing subsidies become available for health plans purchased through the PPACA exchanges and the PPACA Medicaid expansion takes effect, the costs for health coverage and the health plan options at that time will change for individuals who are currently participating in or who were potentially eligible for the HCTC. You asked us to examine issues related to the expiration of the HCTC and its interaction with the PPACA premium tax credit, cost-sharing subsidies, and expansion of Medicaid. Specifically, this report addresses (1) How the expiration of the HCTC and the implementation of the PPACA premium tax credit, cost-sharing subsidies, and Medicaid expansion will affect HCTC participants and nonparticipants, and (2) how the coverage that will be available for plans purchased through the PPACA exchanges compares to HCTC participants' HCTC-qualified health plans' coverage.

To determine how the expiration of the HCTC and implementation of the PPACA premium tax credit, cost-sharing subsidies, and Medicaid expansion will affect HCTC participants and nonparticipants,[12] we analyzed 2010 IRS HCTC program data and individual tax filer data for HCTC participants, which were the most current data available. For the PPACA premium tax credit and the cost-sharing subsidies, we made projections assuming that HCTC participants would meet many of the key eligibility criteria—namely that they would not be eligible for Medicare or Medicaid and would not be enrolled in health plans in which employers paid for the majority of the premium amounts. Using these data, we determined whether each HCTC participant would be eligible for a PPACA premium tax credit on the basis of their household income[13] and, if eligible, estimated the amount of that PPACA premium tax credit. We compared the estimated PPACA premium tax credit amounts to the estimated HCTC amounts for each participant.[14] We also calculated the percentage of income in 2010 that HCTC participants paid for their share of premiums after the HCTC was applied, and compared these amounts to the estimated percentage of their income they will likely pay for premiums with the PPACA premium tax credit assuming their incomes would remain constant. We also used these data to estimate the percentage of HCTC participants who will likely be eligible for PPACA cost-sharing subsidies and the number and percentage of participants who will likely be eligible for Medicaid, depending in part on whether or not their state expands Medicaid. We excluded from our analyses any participants and nonparticipants aged 65 or older at any point in 2010 because they would have likely been eligible for

Medicare and therefore ineligible for either the HCTC, a PPACA premium tax credit, or PPACA cost-sharing subsidies. We conducted the same analyses for HCTC nonparticipants as we did for the HCTC participants using 2010 IRS data.[15] However, we did not make the same assumption that most nonparticipants would meet many of the key eligibility criteria for the PPACA premium tax credit or cost-sharing subsidies because we could not determine why these individuals did not participate in the HCTC. For example, nonparticipants may have been enrolled in health plans paid for by an employer, which would make them ineligible for a PPACA premium tax credit or cost-sharing subsidy. In light of this, our ability to draw conclusions based on our analysis of the data on HCTC nonparticipants was more limited than it was for HCTC participants. We also reviewed regulations, guidance, and selected literature on the PPACA premium tax credit and cost-sharing subsidies. To determine the reliability of IRS's 2010 HCTC program data and individual tax filer data, we reviewed relevant documentation, conducted interviews with IRS officials knowledgeable about the data, and conducted electronic testing of the data to identify obvious errors or outliers. We determined that the data were sufficiently reliable for purposes of this report.

To determine how the coverage that will be available through the PPACA exchanges compares to the qualified health plans for HCTC participants for each HCTC plan type—COBRA, HCTC state-qualified, VEBA, and individual market—we compared the services that plans purchased through the PPACA exchanges will cover, and actuarial values that plans will be offered at through the exchanges, to the services and actuarial values of HCTC-qualified plans. Since COBRA plans are an extension of employer-sponsored health plans, we based our comparison on existing data on the services covered by,[16] and the actuarial values of, employer-sponsored health plans.[17] For HCTC state-qualified plans, we used 2011 IRS HCTC program data to select a nongeneralizable sample of four states to compare the services covered by the plans that will likely be available through the PPACA exchanges in those states, and the actuarial values at which plans will be offered through the exchanges, to the services covered by and the actuarial values of, selected HCTC state-qualified plans.[18] The four states selected—California, Michigan, North Carolina, and Ohio—were among the states with the largest number in 2011 of both individuals potentially eligible for the HCTC and HCTC monthly participants; were geographically varied; and offered different types of HCTC state-qualified plans.[19] In each state we identified the state's likely EHB benchmark plan and the HCTC state-qualified plan with the largest enrollment for our comparison.[20] In California and Michigan we used the benchmark plans that those states selected, and in the other two states we used the largest small group health plan in each state as the potential exchange benchmark plan because HHS has proposed this as the default exchange benchmark if the state does not choose a benchmark plan.[21] In certain states, choosing an existing small group health plan as a benchmark may lead to lower costs for the state than if it chose a different plan.[22]

In the four states, we reviewed health plan documents and interviewed health plan officials from the four potential exchange benchmark plans and the four selected HCTC state-qualified plans.[23] For VEBA plans, we analyzed the HCTC data from the selected states to identify the VEBA plan that had the largest number of HCTC participants. We reviewed health plan documents and interviewed health plan officials for the selected VEBA plan and compared the services covered by the potential exchange benchmark for the state that contained the majority of the VEBA plan's HCTC enrollees to the services covered by the VEBA plan.

We also compared the actuarial values at which plans will be offered through the exchanges to the actuarial value of the VEBA plan. For individual market plans, we used available data on this type of plan to compare the services covered by,[24] and the actuarial value of, plans purchased through the PPACA exchanges to individual market plans.[25] We also reviewed regulations and guidance on EHB, actuarial value, and other insurance market reforms that may affect premiums and cost-sharing in 2014.

To determine the reliability of IRS's 2011 HCTC program data, we reviewed relevant documentation, interviewed officials knowledgeable about the data, and conducted electronic testing of the data to identify obvious errors or outliers. To assess the reliability of the available data on employer-sponsored health plans and individual market health plans, we reviewed the methodologies used to collect and report these data.

Using these methods, we determined that the data were sufficiently reliable for the purposes of this report. We conducted this performance audit from November 2011 to November 2012 in accordance with generally accepted government auditing standards.

Those standards require that we plan and perform the audit to obtain sufficient, appropriate evidence to provide a reasonable basis for our findings and conclusions based on our audit objectives. We believe that the evidence obtained provides a reasonable basis for our findings and conclusions based on our audit objectives.

Background

The HCTC, which pays a portion of health plan premiums for certain eligible workers and retirees, is set to expire at the end of 2013 when certain PPACA provisions, including PPACA premium tax credits, cost-sharing subsidies, and expansion of Medicaid eligibility, are implemented.

HCTC

The HCTC program is administered by the IRS and currently pays for 72.5 percent of health plan premiums for HCTC participants. The amount of the credit is based solely on the participant's health plan premium amount and is not based on other factors, such as the participant's income. As an example of the credit, an HCTC participant with an annual premium of $10,000 would receive a credit of $7,250. Individuals potentially eligible for the HCTC include manufacturing and service workers who lost their jobs due to foreign import competition and were eligible for TAA benefits (representing about 51 percent of all potentially eligible individuals),[26] and certain retirees between the ages of 55 and 64 whose pensions from a former employer were terminated and are now paid by the PBGC (representing about 47 percent of all potentially eligible individuals).[27]

We have previously reported that many potentially eligible individuals do not participate in the HCTC program. In 2010, less than 10 percent of those potentially eligible for the program participated in the HCTC (see table 1). Some of the potentially eligible individuals may in fact not be eligible for the HCTC, for example if they are eligible for Medicare or Medicaid, or if they are covered by their spouse's employer-sponsored health plan under certain conditions. Others may choose not to participate, for example if even with the HCTC they still cannot afford the cost of their share of health plan premiums.

Table 1. Total Number of 2010 HCTC Participants and Nonparticipants

Participation category	Number of individuals
Number of HCTC participants	43,864
Number of HCTC nonparticipants	469,168
Total number of potentially eligible individuals	513,032

Source: GAO analysis of IRS data.

HCTC participants obtain coverage from HCTC-qualified health plans, which include COBRA plans,[28] HCTC state-qualified plans,[29] VEBA plans,[30] and individual market plans.[31] In 2011, the majority of HCTC participants received coverage from COBRA plans (46 percent) or HCTC state-qualified plans (37 percent).[32] A smaller proportion of HCTC participants received coverage from VEBA plans (10 percent) or individual market plans (1 percent).[33]

Selected PPACA Provisions

Beginning on January 1, 2014, a premium tax credit will be available to help eligible tax filers and their dependents pay for qualified health plans purchased through the PPACA exchanges, to be administered by the IRS.[34] PPACA premium tax credits will be calculated using income reported on tax returns.[35] The credits will generally be available to eligible tax filers and their dependents who are (1) enrolled in one or more qualified health plans through a PPACA exchange, and (2) not eligible for minimum essential coverage other than coverage in the individual market.[36] For example, individuals would not be eligible if they had coverage in a government program, such as Medicare or Medicaid, or certain employer-sponsored coverage.[37]

Tax filers eligible for PPACA premium tax credits will be those with household incomes from 100 percent to 400 percent of the federal poverty level (FPL) for the tax year in which they are receiving the PPACA premium tax credit.[38] The amount of the PPACA premium tax credit will vary by household income level, family size, and other factors. It will subsidize a portion of the tax filer's health insurance premiums.[39] The tax filer's contribution to premiums will be based on their household income relative to the FPL, and will range from 2 percent of their household income for those with household incomes from 100 percent to less than133 percent of the FPL, to 9.5 percent of household income for those with household incomes from 300 percent up to 400 percent of the FPL (see table 2).

Eligibility for PPACA premium tax credits by household income level based on the FPL may vary by state because states may choose not to expand eligibility for Medicaid to nonelderly individuals whose household income does not exceed 133 percent of the FPL.[40] Under the PPACA rule, tax filers with household incomes from 100 percent of the FPL and up to 400 percent of the FPL will be eligible for PPACA premium tax credits. However, also under the PPACA rule, in states that expand Medicaid, individuals with household incomes from 100 percent and up to 138 percent of the FPL will be eligible for Medicaid and therefore ineligible for PPACA premium tax credits. Further, in states that do not expand Medicaid, individuals with household incomes from 100 percent and up to 400 percent of the FPL will be eligible for PPACA premium tax credits, and individuals with household incomes less than 100 percent of the FPL will not be eligible for PPACA premium tax credits and may not be eligible for Medicaid, depending on their states' Medicaid eligibility criteria.[41]

Table 2. For Individuals Eligible for PPACA Premium Tax Credits, the Percentage of Household Income That Will Be Spent on Health Care Premiums for Plans Purchased through PPACA Exchanges in 2014

Household income level based on FPL (percent of FPL)	Percentage of income spent on health care premiums (percent of household income)
100 percent to less than 133%	2.0%
At least 133 but less than 150	3.0–4.0
At least 150 but less than 200	4.0–6.3
At least 200 but less than 250	6.3–8.05
At least 250 but less than 300	8.05–9.5
At least 300 and up to 400	9.5

Source: IRS and 26 C.F.R. §§ 1.36B-2(b), 1.36B-3(g)(2) (2012).

The applicable household income level expressed as a percent of the FPL determines an individual's share of his or her annual premium. The amount of the premium for the second-lowest-cost silver plan in the PPACA exchange available in the state where the eligible individual resides will be the reference for calculating the amount of the PPACA premium tax credit.[42] See table 3 for an example of a PPACA premium tax credit for two different people, both in a family of four, one with a household income at 150 percent of the FPL, and the other with a household income at 300 percent of the FPL, using a hypothetical annual premium of $10,000 for the second-lowest-cost silver plan (reference plan) in the PPACA exchange available in the state where they reside.

Enrollees may also be eligible for separate, PPACA cost-sharing subsidies to help reduce their out-of-pocket expenses such as deductibles and copays.[43] However, as with the PPACA premium tax credits, tax filers will not be eligible for PPACA cost-sharing subsidies if they are eligible for Medicaid in their state. PPACA cost-sharing subsidies will reduce the maximum out-of-pocket limit for eligible individuals (not including health plan premiums).[44] For example, had the limits been in place in 2010, an eligible individual with an income of 150 percent of the FPL would have had his or her maximum out-of-pocket limit reduced by two-thirds. Therefore, the individual's maximum out-of-pocket limit would have been about $1,981 instead of $5,950 for single coverage.

Table 3. Example of a PPACA Premium Tax Credit in 2014 at Two Different Income Levels Based on a Hypothetical Reference Plan with a Premium of $10,000

			Tax filer's share for annual premium amount	
Household income (percentage of FPL)	**Hypothetical annual premium amount**	**Annual PPACA premium tax credit**	**Percentage of household income**	**Dollar amount**
$33,075 (150% FPL)	$10,000	$8,677	4%	$1,323
66,150 (300)	10,000	3,716	9.5	6,284

Source: GAO.

Note: Example is based on 2010 FPLs for the contiguous 48 states and the District of Columbia for a family size of four.

PPACA Exchanges

PPACA provides for the establishment and operation of exchanges in each state that will provide competitive marketplaces for qualified individuals[45] and small employers[46] to directly compare and purchase available private health insurance plans by January 1, 2014.[47]

PPACA requires that health plans purchased through the PPACA exchanges offer services in each of the following EHB categories:

- ambulatory patient services;
- emergency services;
- hospitalization;
- maternity and newborn care;
- mental health and substance use disorder services, including behavioral health treatment;
- prescription drugs;
- rehabilitative and habilitative services and devices;

- laboratory services;
- preventive and wellness services and chronic disease management; and
- pediatric services, including oral and vision care.

CCIIO will oversee the implementation and operation of the exchanges, including the provision of guidance on EHB categories and the actuarial value of plans purchased through the PPACA exchanges. Because each state will have its own benchmark plan, EHB services may vary by state.[48] Health plans will be offered at four levels of actuarial value through the exchanges and designated by different metal tiers. These levels of coverage will allow individuals purchasing a plan to compare what the potential differences in out-of-pocket expenses would be for each plan. The four metal tiers include the following:

- bronze: plans that have actuarial values of 60 percent,
- silver: plans that have actuarial values of 70 percent,
- gold: plans that have actuarial values of 80 percent, and
- platinum: plans that have actuarial values of 90 percent.[49]

When the HCTC Expires Most HCTC Participants Will Likely Be Ineligible for a PPACA Premium Tax Credit or Eligible for a Credit Less Generous Than the HCTC

The expiration of the HCTC and implementation of the PPACA premium tax credits and Medicaid expansion will affect HCTC participants' costs for health plans in multiple ways. Projections from our analysis of 2010 IRS data show that about 69 percent of HCTC participants will likely either be ineligible for a PPACA premium tax credit or Medicaid, or will be eligible for a PPACA premium tax credit that is less generous than the HCTC. These projections show that about 37 percent of HCTC participants will likely be ineligible for either a PPACA premium tax credit or Medicaid because their incomes are too high, and 32 percent will be eligible for a PPACA premium tax credit less generous than the HCTC. On the other hand, at least 27 percent of HCTC participants will be eligible for a PPACA premium tax credit more generous than the HCTC or be eligible for Medicaid. An additional 3 percent of all participants will likely be ineligible for a PPACA premium tax credit because their incomes are too low, and their eligibility for Medicaid will depend in part on their state's decision on Medicaid expansion (see table 4).

Table 4. Percentage of HCTC Participants Who Will Likely Be Eligible and Ineligible for a PPACA Premium Tax Credit, and Possibly Eligible for Medicaid in 2014

HCTC participants	Number	Percentage (among all HCTC participants)
Eligible for PPACA premium tax credit (household income >138% FPL to 400% FPL)	21,748	55%
Credit more generous than HCTC	9,054[a]	23
Credit less generous than HCTC	12,694[a]	32
Either eligible for PPACA premium tax credit more generous than HCTC[b] or eligible for Medicaid (household income 100% FPL to 138% FPL)	1,678[a]	4
Ineligible for PPACA premium tax credit but possibly eligible for Medicaid (household income <100% FPL)	1,312	3
Ineligible for PPACA premium tax credit (household income >400% FPL)	14,726	37
Total number of participants	39,464[c]	100%

Source: GAO analysis of IRS data.

Notes: The percentages may not add to 100 percent because of rounding.

[a]To compare the PPACA premium tax credit amounts to the HCTC amounts, we calculated PPACA premium tax credits using the same premium amount each HCTC participant was estimated to have paid for his or her HCTC coverage.

[b]For participants who will likely be eligible for a PPACA premium tax credit because their state did not expand Medicaid, the tax credit will likely be more generous than the HCTC.

[c]We excluded all participants who were age 65 or older in 2010, and those for whom we were unable to obtain tax data. As a result, 39,464 of the 43,864 participants in 2010 were included in our analyses.

For the HCTC participants who will likely be eligible for a PPACA premium tax credit in 2014, projections from our analysis of 2010 IRS data show that there will be variation in the extent to which their credit differs from the HCTC. For example, of the total 39,464 HCTC participants in our analysis, 6,492 will likely receive a PPACA premium tax credit at least 25 percent less than the HCTC. However, up to 12,141 participants will likely receive a credit similar to or greater than the HCTC. For example, 2,922 participants will likely receive a PPACA premium tax credit of about the same value as the HCTC (within 5 percentage points above or below the HCTC). In addition, depending in part on whether or not their state expands Medicaid, between 1,823 and 3,217 participants will likely receive a credit more than 25 percent higher than the HCTC (see fig. 1).

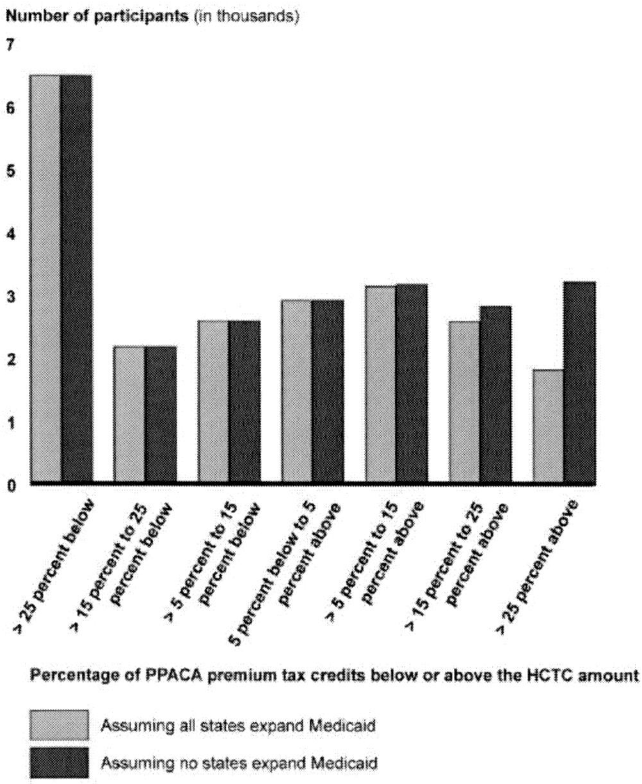

Source: GAO analysis of IRS data.

Note: To compare the PPACA premium tax credit amounts to the HCTC amounts, we calculated PPACA premium tax credits using the same premium amount each HCTC participant was estimated to have paid for his or her HCTC coverage.

Figure 1. Comparison of the PPACA Premium Tax Credit to the HCTC among HCTC Participants Who Will Likely Be Eligible for a PPACA Premium Tax Credit in 2014.

The PPACA premium tax credit was designed to provide a larger subsidy amount to lower-income tax filers than to higher-income tax filers. Thus, lower-income HCTC participants who will likely be eligible for a PPACA premium tax credit[50] will pay a smaller share of their incomes for premiums under PPACA in 2014 than they did under the HCTC.

For example, projections from our analysis of 2010 IRS data show that while all 2,488 HCTC participants with incomes from 100 percent[51] to 150 percent of the FPL will likely pay between 2 percent and 4 percent of their incomes for health plan premiums under the PPACA rule, 1,456 HCTC participants—close to 60 percent of participants in the same income range—paid 9.5 percent or more of their incomes for health plan premiums under the HCTC. In contrast, while all 7,658 HCTC participants with incomes from 300 percent to 400 percent of the FPL[52] will likely pay 9.5 percent of their household income for premiums under the PPACA rule, 2,391—over 30 percent of participants in the same income range— paid less than 4 percent of their household income for premiums under the HCTC (see fig. 2). Unlike the HCTC that pays 72.5 percent of health plan premiums, individuals eligible for a PPACA premium tax credit will continue to pay that set percentage even if premiums increase because PPACA rules limit the amount individuals will pay for premiums to a set percentage of their incomes.[53]

The expiration of the HCTC and implementation of PPACA cost-sharing subsidies will also affect HCTC participants' out-of-pocket costs for health plans. Projections from our analysis of 2010 IRS data show that up to 28 percent of all HCTC participants who are eligible for the PPACA premium tax credit will likely also be eligible for a PPACA cost-sharing subsidy in 2014 to help pay for deductibles and copays, depending in part on whether or not their state expands Medicaid. Similar cost-sharing subsidies are not available for the HCTC, therefore, this would be an additional financial benefit for those who qualify.

The effect of the expiration of the HCTC and implementation of certain PPACA provisions will likely be different for nonparticipants[54]—individuals who were potentially eligible for the HCTC in 2010 but did not participate in it—than it will be for participants. First, nonparticipants who may not be eligible for PPACA premium tax credits or who may be eligible for tax credits less generous than the HCTC will not be losing any benefits because they are not receiving the HCTC. Our projections show that 70 percent of nonparticipants fall into this category. Second, because some individuals do not participate in the HCTC since they cannot afford to do so, some nonparticipants who will be eligible for PPACA premium tax credits that are more generous than the HCTC or who are eligible for Medicaid coverage under PPACA may choose to use these options and receive benefits they do not receive under the HCTC.

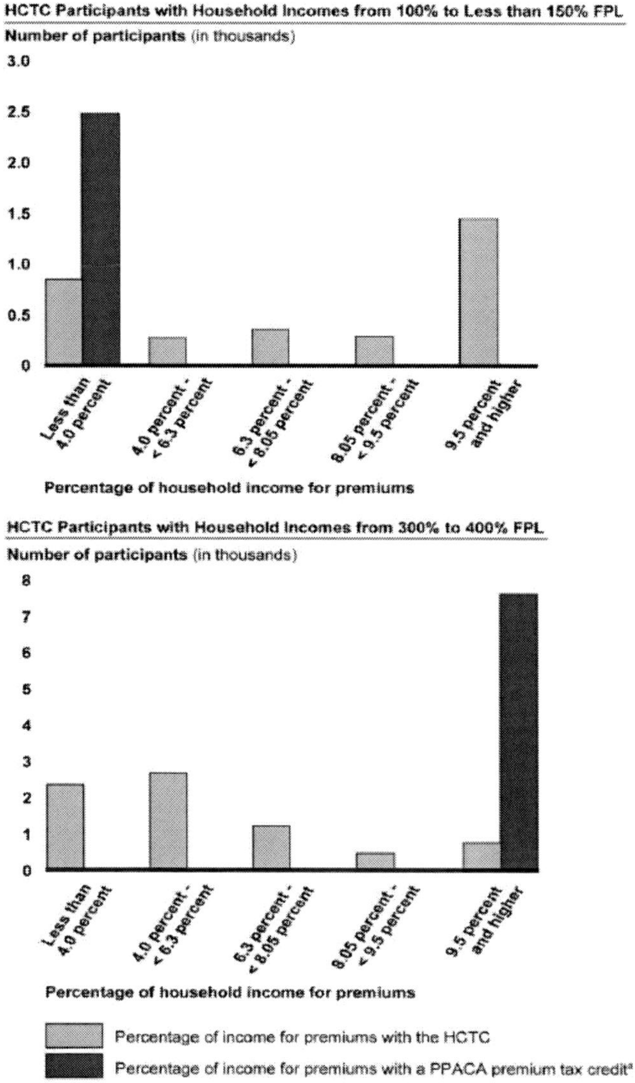

Source: GAO analysis of IRS data.

[a]This analysis assumes that the second-lowest-cost silver plan was chosen. The percentage of household income for premiums with a PPACA premium tax credit may vary if a more or less generous plan is purchased through the exchanges.

Figure 2. Comparison of the Percentage of Household Income Spent on Premiums with the HCTC to Premiums with a PPACA Premium Tax Credit among HCTC Participants Who Will Likely Be Eligible for a PPACA Premium Tax Credit in 2014.

Our projections show that up to 30 percent of nonparticipants fall into this category, depending in part on whether or not their state expands Medicaid and whether they meet all other eligibility criteria for the PPACA premium tax credits.[55] In addition to being eligible for the PPACA premium tax credit, based on projections from our analysis of 2010 IRS data, up to 30 percent of all HCTC nonparticipants may also be eligible for a PPACA cost-sharing subsidy in 2014 to help pay for deductibles and copays, depending in part on whether or not their state expands Medicaid and whether they meet all other eligibility criteria for the PPACA premium tax credits. See appendix I for details on characteristics of 2010 HCTC participants and nonparticipants.

Health Plan Coverage under PPACA Will Be Comparable to HCTC Plans, but Participants May Have an Incentive to Change Their Level of Coverage

The health plan coverage available under PPACA will be comparable to coverage in current HCTC-qualified health plans. Specifically, the categories of services that plans purchased through the PPACA exchanges will be required to cover are comparable to those currently covered by most HCTC plans, and the actuarial values of HCTC plans are likely above the minimum level of coverage that will be required in PPACA exchange plans. However, under PPACA, HCTC participants may have an incentive to choose plans through the exchanges that have different levels of coverage than their HCTC plans.

The Categories of Services That Will Be Required for Plans Purchased through the PPACA Exchanges Are Comparable to the Categories of Services Currently Covered by HCTC Plans

The EHB categories that will be required for plans purchased through the PPACA exchanges are comparable to the categories of services covered in almost all of the health plans used now by HCTC participants. Specifically, the categories covered by COBRA plans as well as the four HCTC state-qualified plans and the VEBA plan that we reviewed are comparable to the EHB categories. Collectively, at least 93 percent of HCTC participants in 2011 were enrolled in these three types of HCTC plans. However, for two of the EHB categories—"rehabilitative and habilitative services and devices" and "pediatric services, including oral and vision care"—more services may be covered by the plans purchased through the PPACA exchanges than are covered by the COBRA, HCTC state-qualified, and VEBA plans. This is because many health plans, whether HCTC or other, do not currently cover habilitative services or pediatric dental and vision services. While not all of the EHB categories are covered by individual market plans, only about 1 percent of HCTC participants are covered by individual market plans.

COBRA Plans (46 Percent of HCTC Participants)

COBRA plans are an extension of employer-sponsored health plans, and our analysis of data reported in a 2011 Department of Labor report found that employer-sponsored health plans generally covered services in the EHB categories.[56] For example, in the EHB category of ambulatory care, 100 percent of employer-sponsored health plans cover physician office visits; 98 percent of plans cover outpatient surgery; and 73 percent of plans cover home health care services. In addition, the report indicated that the majority of employer-sponsored health plans cover services in the EHB categories of hospitalization, emergency services, maternity care, mental health and substance abuse disorders, and prescription drugs. Although COBRA plans generally cover services in the EHB categories, it is possible that coverage of habilitative services and pediatric dental and vision services will be more generous in plans purchased through the PPACA exchanges than in COBRA plans. According to CCIIO, the EHB categories that are commonly not covered among typical employer plans are habilitative services, pediatric oral services, and pediatric vision services.[57]

HCTC State-Qualified Plans (37 Percent of HCTC Participants)

Our analysis of four 2012 HCTC state-qualified plans found that they also generally covered services in all of the EHB categories. Specifically, all of the plans we reviewed—including both the four potential exchange benchmark plans and the four HCTC state-qualified plans—covered services in the same EHB categories, such as ambulatory care, preventive care, laboratory services, hospitalization, and emergency services. In addition, all of the plans covered prescription drugs to some extent; although one of the HCTC state-qualified plans that we reviewed covered generic prescriptions but did not cover brand-name prescriptions. Among some of the HCTC state-qualified plans and the potential benchmark plans there was an absence of coverage for subsets of services in certain EHB categories, such as habilitative services and pediatric dental and vision services, which are services that will be required to be covered in plans sold through the PPACA exchanges. For example, habilitative services were not covered by two of the potential exchange benchmark plans or by three of the HCTC state-qualified plans.[58]

VEBA Plans (10 Percent of HCTC Participants)

The potential exchange benchmark plans cover the same EHB categories that the 2012 VEBA plan that we reviewed does. Also, like some of the potential exchange benchmark plans, the VEBA plan does not cover certain services that are a subset of certain EHB categories, such as habilitative services.

Individual Market Plans (1 Percent of HCTC Participants)

Plans purchased through the PPACA exchanges may provide coverage of EHB categories in which coverage may be more limited in individual market plans. In 2011, HHS reported that coverage of certain EHB categories is limited in individual market plans, specifically for maternity services, substance abuse services, mental health services, and prescription drugs.[59] However, only about 1 percent of HCTC participants are enrolled in individual market plans.

HCTC Plans' Actuarial Values Are Likely above PPACA's Minimum Level of Value

The vast majority of HCTC participants in 2012 were likely enrolled in plans with actuarial values that were above the minimum level of 60 percent (bronze) required for plans purchased through the PPACA exchanges, including many who were likely enrolled in plans that had actuarial values of 80 percent (gold) or higher.

COBRA Plans (46 Percent of HCTC Participants)

The majority of HCTC participants in COBRA plans are likely to be in plans with actuarial values of 80 percent or higher on the basis of data from two studies. One study estimated that 80 percent of all enrollees in employer-sponsored health plans in 2010 were in plans that met or exceeded 80 percent (gold).[60] The other study estimated that about 65 percent of all employees enrolled in group health plans in 2010 were in plans with actuarial values that met or exceeded 80 percent (gold).[61]

HCTC State-Qualified and VEBA Plans (47 Percent of HCTC Participants Combined)

The actuarial values of the four HCTC state-qualified plans and the one VEBA plan that we reviewed in the selected states vary. However, all of the plans have an actuarial value of at least 60 percent (bronze) and three of the five plans have an actuarial value of 80 percent (gold) or higher.[62] See table 5.

Table 5. Actuarial Value of Selected HCTC Plans in Selected States, 2012

			Actuarial value level of coverage (percent)[b]		
Selected HCTC plan[a]	**Below 60**	**60–69**	**70-79**	**80-89**	**Above 90**
Plan 1					X
Plan 2		X			
Plan 3[c]		X			
Plan 4				X	
Plan 5					X
Total	**0**	**2**	**0**	**1**	**2**

Source: GAO analysis of interviews with health plan officials.

[a]The five selected plans include four HCTC state-qualified plans and one VEBA plan. Plan officials provided all actuarial values during interviews with GAO. All values reflect the plan coverage available in 2012 with the exception of Plan 3's value.

[b]For the purposes of our analysis, we used actuarial value ranges of 10 percentage points for each level of coverage. Plan officials told us the actuarial value range that each plan was in (i.e. 70- 79 percent) rather than the specific actuarial value estimate. However, HHS has proposed a de *minimis* variation of +/-2 percentage points (e.g., a silver-level plan will be able to have a value from 68 to 72 percent) in actuarial value rather than the wider range of actuarial values at each level of coverage that our analysis used. CCIIO officials told us that plans that have actuarial values that do not fall within +/-2 percentage points of one of the levels of coverage will not be sold inside or outside of an exchange.

[c]Plan 3's actuarial value was calculated using estimated 2010 costs and utilization for the plan's standard population rather than estimated costs and utilization for the current (2012) standard population of the plan. A plan official told us that it is likely that actuarial value has increased slightly since 2010, as the plan's deductibles have not increased since 2010 to accommodate any increases in inflation.

Individual Market Plans (1 Percent of HCTC Participants)

The small number of HCTC participants that have individual market plans are likely to have a plan with a lower level of actuarial value. A recent study[63] found that about half of the plans (51 percent) in the individual market have an actuarial value of less than 60 percent and another third (33 percent) have an actuarial value at the 60 percent (bronze) level.[64]

Certain PPACA Provisions May Incentivize HCTC Participants to Change Their Level of Coverage in 2014

The varied actuarial values of the HCTC plans suggest that the level of coverage for many HCTC participants may change after the expiration of the HCTC depending on the options available to participants and the choices they make in 2014 under PPACA. Also, the way that the PPACA tax credits will be calculated may incentivize HCTC participants to change their level of coverage.[65] The PPACA premium tax credits will be calculated from a reference plan at the 70 percent (silver) level of coverage, so individuals who choose other plans—with either higher or lower levels of actuarial value—could face higher or lower out-of-pocket costs for premiums. However, plans with higher levels of actuarial value may result in lower out-of-pocket costs for copays and deductibles, and plans with lower levels of actuarial value may result in higher out-of-pocket costs for copays and deductibles. Ultimately, for any HCTC participant, the overall financial effect of a change from an HCTC plan to a PPACA exchange plan will be the net effect of the choice between higher or lower premium costs and higher or lower cost-sharing.[66] Further, out-of-pocket costs for premiums and cost-sharing for HCTC participants will be affected by whether they are eligible for the PPACA premium tax credits and cost-sharing subsidies.[67] Considering these factors, current HCTC participants may choose to change their level of coverage when the HCTC expires. For example:

- **Some HCTC participants eligible for PPACA premium tax credits could have an incentive to change to a higher level of coverage**. For example, if the HCTC participants who have coverage at the 60 percent (bronze) level of coverage are eligible for PPACA premium tax credits, they may choose a PPACA exchange plan that has a higher actuarial value than their current HCTC plan. This is because PPACA premium tax credit amounts will be calculated on the basis of the reference plan premium (the second-lowest-cost 70 percent [silver] plan) for their exchange. Given this, it could be possible for these HCTC participants to purchase a 70 percent (silver) plan that would have on average lower out-of-pocket cost-sharing expenses than their current HCTC plan.

- **Alternatively, some HCTC participants who will be eligible for PPACA premium tax credits could have an incentive to change to a lower level of coverage**. For example, if the HCTC participants who have coverage at the 80 percent (gold) or 90 percent (platinum) levels of coverage are eligible for a PPACA premium tax credit and want to purchase a plan through a PPACA exchange with a comparable actuarial value, they will have to pay the difference between the premium for a plan with an actuarial value of 80 percent (gold) or 90 percent (platinum) and their PPACA premium tax credit. Again, this is because the PPACA premium tax credit amount will be based on the reference plan premium (the second-lowest-cost 70 percent [silver] plan) for their exchange. For example, if a participant in a family of four with a household income at 300 percent of the FPL purchases a plan in a PPACA exchange with an annual reference (silver) plan premium for a family of four of $10,000, he or she would receive a PPACA premium tax credit of $3,716 and would have to pay $6,284 for the premium if he or she purchased the reference plan. However, if the participant instead decided to purchase a plan with an actuarial value of 80 percent (gold) having an annual premium of $11,000, the PPACA premium tax credit would remain the same ($3,716) but the premium amount the participant would have to pay would increase by $1,000 to $7,284. Because participants would have to pay this difference in premiums, they may opt to purchase a plan with a lower level of actuarial value than their current plan, such as a plan at the 70 percent level of coverage (silver), even though it may have higher out-of-pocket cost-sharing expenses on average than their current plan.

  In contrast, HCTC participants may also have an incentive to choose a plan below the 70 percent (silver) level if obtaining the lowest possible premium is their main factor in choosing a health plan.

  In this case, participants could choose a plan at the 60 percent (bronze) level of coverage because the premium cost would likely be lower than choosing a 70 percent (silver) level plan. However, a plan at this level would mean that on average participants could have higher out-of-pocket cost-sharing expenses than they would with a 70 percent (silver) plan.

- **The health plan coverage options for HCTC participants not eligible for a PPACA premium tax credit will vary depending on their household income level.** The HCTC participants' not eligible for PPACA premium tax credits because their incomes are above 400 percent of the FPL could decide to purchase a health plan at any level of coverage.

  However, the loss of the HCTC combined with their ineligibility for PPACA premium tax credits because of their higher incomes could affect the level of coverage that they choose or even whether they purchase a health plan through a PPACA exchange or elsewhere.

  The HCTC participants who have household incomes below 138 percent of the FPL and live in states that expand Medicaid will not be eligible for PPACA premium tax credits; instead they will be eligible for Medicaid.

  However, in states that do not expand Medicaid, it is uncertain what health plan, if any, that HCTC participants who have household incomes below 100 percent of the FPL may purchase in 2014. These individuals would not be eligible for PPACA premium tax credit in any instance or Medicaid in most instances, and their ability to pay for premiums will be limited.

  However, because of their low incomes, these HCTC participants will likely be exempt from certain PPACA provisions, such as the tax penalty that individuals will have to pay beginning in 2014 if they do not have a health plan.[68]

AGENCY COMMENTS

We provided draft copies of this report to HHS and IRS for review, and both provided technical comments, which we incorporated as appropriate.

John E. Dicken
Director,
Health Care

APPENDIX I: CHARACTERISTICS OF HEALTH COVERAGE TAX CREDIT (HCTC) PARTICIPANTS AND NONPARTICIPANTS IN 2010

We identified HCTC participants and nonparticipants by age groups, household income based on a percentage of the federal poverty level (FPL), and HCTC eligibility type using 2010 Internal Revenue Service (IRS) data.

Table 6. Number and Percentage of HCTC Participants and Nonparticipants by Age Groups in 2010

	Participants[a]	Nonparticipants[a]		
	Number	Percent	Number	Percent
34 or younger	1,127	3%	31,577	8%
35–44	3,505	9	48,462	13
45–54	8,370	22	70,316	19
55–64	24,733	66	223,878	60

Source: GAO analysis of IRS data.

[a]This analysis excludes all participants and nonparticipants who were age 65 or older in 2010, any tax filers for whom we could not identify an age, and those for whom we were unable to obtain tax data. As a result, 86 percent of participants and 80 percent of nonparticipants were included in this analysis.

Table 7. Number and Percentage of HCTC Participants and Nonparticipants by Household Income Based on the FPL in 2010

Household income by percent of FPL	Participants[a]		Nonparticipants[a]	
	Number	Percent	Number	Percent
<100%	1,312	3%	25,935	7%
100 to <150	2,488	6	38,003	10
150 to <200	4,205	11	42,512	11
200 to <250	4,424	11	38,457	10
250 to <300	4,651	12	36,972	10
300 to 400	7,658	19	65,022	17
>400	14,726	37	143,302	37

Source: GAO analysis of IRS data.

Notes: The percentages may not add to 100 percent because of rounding.

[a]This analysis excludes all participants and nonparticipants who were age 65 or older in 2010, and those for whom we were unable to obtain tax data. As a result, 90 percent of participants and 83 percent of nonparticipants were included in this analysis.

We found that most HCTC participants and nonparticipants were ages 55 to 64 (see table 6), over a third of participants and nonparticipants had household income greater than 400 percent of the FPL (see table 7), and more than half were potentially eligible for the HCTC because of participation in the Trade Adjustment Assistance (TAA) or Reemployment Trade Adjustment Assistance (RTAA) programs rather than being eligible by having their pension payments assumed by the Pension Benefit Guaranty Corporation (PBGC) (see table 8).

Table 8. Number and Percentage of HCTC Participants and Nonparticipants by Eligibility Type in 2010

	Participants[a]		Nonparticipants[a]	
Eligibility Type	**Number**	**Percent**	**Number**	**Percent**
TAA or RTAA	22,148	59	214,843	55
PBGC	14,443	38	170,458	44
Multiple Eligibility[b]	1,136	3	4,898	1

Source: GAO analysis of IRS data.

[a]This analysis excludes all participants and nonparticipants who were age 65 or older in 2010, any tax filers for whom we could not identify an eligibility type, and those for whom we were unable to obtain tax data. As a result, 86 percent of participants and 83 percent of nonparticipants were included in this analysis.

[b]According to IRS officials, HCTC participants and nonparticipants may have multiple eligibility types, for example, individuals may be eligible through TAA benefits and by having their pension payments assumed by PBGC.

End Notes

[1] Pub. L. No. 107-210, div. A, § 201, 116 Stat. 935, 954. The HCTC was applicable to tax years beginning in 2002.

[2] Pub. L. No. 112-40, title II, § 241, 125 Stat. 402, 418. The increased credit rate was applicable to coverage months beginning after February 12, 2011.

[3] *See* Pub. L. No. 111-148, title I, subtitles D and E, title X, subtitle A, §§ 10104, and 10105, 124 Stat. 119, 162, 213, 896, 906 (2010), as amended by the Health Care and Education Reconciliation Act of 2010, Pub. L. No. 111-152, title I, subtitle A, 124 Stat. 1029, 1030. For purposes of this report, references to PPACA include the amendments made by the Health Care and Education Reconciliation Act of 2010.

[4] An exchange is a mechanism for organizing the health insurance marketplace to help consumers and small businesses shop for health insurance plans and compare available plan options based on price, benefits, and quality. Throughout this report we refer to these as PPACA exchanges.

[5] Pub. L. No. 111-148, §§ 2001, 10201(c), 124 Stat. 271, 1051, as amended by Pub. L. No. 111-152 § 1201, 124 Stat. 1051. Eligibility for Medicaid varies by state. However, in most

states, nondisabled childless adults are not currently eligible for Medicaid regardless of age or level of income. Under the Medicaid program, failure by a state to comply with federal requirements may result in a termination of federal Medicaid matching funds. However, the U.S. Supreme Court has ruled that states choosing not to expand Medicaid coverage to this group of individuals will forgo only the federal matching funds associated with such expanded coverage. See National Federation of Independent Business, et al., vs. Sebelius, Sec. of Health and Human Services, et al., 567 U.S. ___, 2012 WL 2427810 (U.S. June 28, 2012).

[6] See GAO, *Health Coverage Tax Credit: Participation and Administrative Costs*, GAO-10-521R (Washington, D.C.: Apr. 30, 2010).

[7] There are several reasons why individuals who are identified as potentially eligible may ultimately be ineligible for the HCTC. One reason is that HCTC eligibility is conditioned on the individual not having "other specified coverage," which is defined to include coverage under Medicare, Medicaid, or the state Children's Health Insurance Program. 26 U.S.C. § 35 (b)(1)(A)(iii), (f). Medicare is the federally financed health care program for persons 65 years of age or over as well as for certain individuals with disabilities and individuals with end-stage renal disease. Medicaid and the state Children's Health Insurance Program are joint federal-state programs that finance health care for certain categories of low-income individuals.

[8] 26 U.S.C. § 35(a), (e).

[9] VEBAs may be established through bankruptcy court to provide certain specified benefits, including group health benefits, and are generally similar to employer-sponsored health plans. Group coverage obtained through a spouse's current or former employer may also be HCTC-qualified, with certain restrictions.

[10] Pub. L. No. 111-148, §§ 1301, 1302, 1311, 1321, 10104, 124 Stat. 162, 163, 173, 186, 896.

[11] Pub. L. No. 111-148, §§ 1302 (d (2), 10104(b)(1), 124 Stat. 167, 896. Accordingly, the actuarial value of a plan represents the expected percentage of costs the plan will incur for the EHB services provided to a standard population. For example, a gold plan with an 80 percent actuarial value would be expected to pay, on average, 80 percent of a standard population's expected medical expenses for the EHB. The individuals covered by the plan would be expected to pay, on average, the remaining 20 percent of the expected cost-sharing expenses in the form of deductibles, copayments, and coinsurance.

[12] For the purposes of our analysis we assumed that individuals in all states could potentially be eligible for PPACA premium tax credits, consistent with the final rule issued by IRS. *See* Health Insurance Premium Tax Credit, preamble 1.f and regulations to be codified at 26 C.F.R. §§ 1.36B-0 et seq., 77 Fed. Reg. 30377, 30378, 30385 (May 23, 2012). In addition, we limited our analysis of participants who will likely be eligible for cost-sharing subsidies to those earning up to 250 percent of the federal poverty level (FPL), consistent with CCIIO guidance. See Center for Consumer Information and Insurance Oversight, *Actuarial Value and Cost-Sharing Reductions Bulletin* (Feb. 24, 2012).

[13] Household income was calculated by summing the income of each participant with the incomes of each participant's spouse and dependents.

[14] These estimates are from estimated annualized HCTC premiums for all HCTC participants. Participants can receive the HCTC in two ways: yearly as a tax credit when they file their federal income tax returns, or monthly as an advance payment directly to their health plans when their premiums are due each month. Data on HCTC monthly participants included monthly 2010 HCTC amounts, which we used to calculate annualized HCTC premiums. We calculated an estimated annualized HCTC premium for monthly participants who did

not receive the HCTC for all 12 months in 2010. To calculate the estimated annualized HCTC premiums for yearly participants, we used available data on premium amounts from monthly HCTC participants and calculated a state average in the states in which these monthly participants lived in 2010. The state average estimate was applied to yearly participants according to the state in which they lived in 2010. We also used these estimated annualized HCTC premiums as the basis for our estimation of the PPACA premium tax credit amounts.

[15] We also calculated an estimated annualized HCTC premium for HCTC nonparticipants using available data on premium amounts from monthly HCTC participants in the states in which these monthly participants lived in 2010. The state average estimate was applied to nonparticipants according to the state in which they lived in 2010. We used these estimated annualized HCTC premiums as the basis for our estimation of the PPACA premium tax credit amounts. In addition, we limited our analysis of nonparticipants who will likely be eligible for cost-sharing subsidies to those earning up to 250 percent of the FPL, consistent with the 2012 CCIIO bulletin on cost-sharing reductions.

[16] Department of Labor, *Selected Medical Benefits: A Report From the Department of Labor to the Department of Health and Human Services* (Washington, D.C.: April 2011).

[17] Department of Health and Human Services, Office of the Assistant Secretary for Planning and Evaluation, *Actuarial Value and Employer-Sponsored Insurance* (Washington, D.C.: November 2011).

used 2011 IRS HCTC program data to select the states because 2011 was the most recent year of data available regarding the types of HCTC-qualified plans that participants have.

[19] In 2011, the four selected states combined represented 28 percent of all individuals potentially eligible for the HCTC and 34 percent of all monthly participants. At the time of our analysis, data on yearly participants for 2011 were not yet available, so we selected states with the highest numbers of individuals potentially eligible for the HCTC and monthly participants in 2011.

[20] Throughout this report we refer to these plans as potential exchange benchmark plans.

[21] Patient Protection and Affordable Care Act; Standards Related to Essential Health Benefits, Actuarial Value, and Accreditation, 77 Fed. Reg. 70644, 70670 (proposed Nov. 26, 2011) (to be codified at 45 C.F.R. § 156.100(c)). The term “small group” is used to describe health plans offered by employers with 100 or fewer employees.

[22] States will be required to defray the costs of state-mandated benefits in addition to EHB. *See* Pub. L. No. 111-148, § 1311(d)(3)(B),124 Stat. 176. However, HHS has proposed that a state not be required to defray the costs of state-mandated benefits enacted on or before December 31, 2011 as they would be considered EHB. See, 77 Fed. Reg. 70644, 70647, 70668 (to be codified at 45 C.F.R. § 155.170(a)(2)). Because small group plans are typically subject to many of a state’s mandated benefits, states may be more likely to choose a small group plan as their benchmark plan.

[23] We reviewed health plan documents for the 2012 plan year for the HCTC state-qualified plans and potential exchange benchmark plans which were the most current data available. We also used 2012 plan documents for the VEBA plan we reviewed.

[24] Department of Health and Human Services, Office of the Assistant Secretary for Planning and Evaluation, *Essential Health Benefits: Individual Market Coverage* (Washington, D.C.: December 2011).

[25] Jon.R Gabel et al., “More Than Half of Individual Health Plans Offer Coverage That Falls Short Of What Can Be Sold Through Exchanges As of 2014,” *Health Affairs*, vol. 31, no 6 (Bethesda, Md.: June 2012).

[26] Within the TAA program, there is a Reemployment Trade Adjustment Assistance (RTAA) program. The RTAA program provides a wage subsidy to workers aged 50 years or older who have lost their jobs because of foreign import competition and have accepted a job where they earn less money than they did at their prior job. Throughout this report, any reference to TAA eligible individuals includes both TAA and RTAA eligible individuals.

[27] About 1 percent of individuals potentially eligible for the HCTC have multiple eligibility types—they are eligible both through receiving TAA benefits and because their pensions are now paid by PBGC—and for about less than 1 percent, HCTC eligibility type could not be identified.

[28] COBRA in general requires employers that offer group health plans (i.e., employer-sponsored health plans) and have 20 or more employees to make health insurance available for a limited period of time for employees and their dependents who have lost health insurance because of certain events, including the loss of employment. Former employees who opt to continue their coverage through COBRA are responsible for the full cost of the health plan premium and the administrative costs for the continuation of coverage (not to exceed 102 percent of the applicable premium for such period). *See* 29 U.S.C. §§ 1161-1168.

[29] HCTC state-qualified plans are health plans designated by each state's department of insurance. A state-qualified plan may be a private health insurance plan offered by a company or a public health insurance plan offered by a state (e.g., state high-risk pool). These plans must offer certain statutorily defined consumer protections.

[30] VEBAs may be established for individuals who have an employment-related common bond (e.g., common employer, coverage under one or more collective bargaining agreements, etc.) through a bankruptcy court to provide certain specified benefits, including health benefits, to their members or their members' designated beneficiaries. VEBAs can provide health plan benefits in place of COBRA and retiree benefits. Coverage under a VEBA may receive consideration for HCTC purposes only for eligible coverage months beginning before February 13, 2012.

[31] Group coverage obtained through a spouse's current or former employer may also be HCTC-qualified, with certain restrictions. Certain types of health plans do not qualify for the HCTC, including the Federal Employees Health Benefits plans, stand-alone dental or vision plans, and long-term care benefits; or coverage for only a specified disease or illness. HCTC candidates enrolled in these plans would not be eligible for the HCTC.

[32] Data on the HCTC plan types of the 2011 yearly participants were not available, so all of the percentages are based on the HCTC plan types of the 2011 monthly participants.

[33] About 6 percent of monthly participants in 2011 had multiple types of HCTC plans, which means that they may have changed plans during the year, such as switching from a COBRA plan to a HCTC state-qualified plan.

[34] *See* Pub. L. No. 111-148, title I, subtitles D and E, title X, subtitle A, §§ 10104 and 10105, 124 Stat. 162, 213, 896, 906, as amended by Pub. L. No. 111-152, title I, subtitle A, 124 Stat. 1030. *See* also 26 C.F.R. §§ 1.36B-0 et seq.

[35] Therefore, the PPACA premium tax credits can only be obtained by eligible individuals who file tax returns.

[36] 26 C.F.R. § 1.36B-2 (2012). "Minimum essential coverage" includes health plans such as individual market health plans, eligible employer-sponsored health plans (if they meet affordability and quality standards), or government-sponsored health coverage such as Medicare, Medicaid, and the Children's Health Insurance Program. See 26 U.S.C. § 5000A(f).

[37] PPACA also requires that individuals, subject to certain exceptions, obtain minimum essential health insurance coverage or pay a tax penalty. Pub. L. No. 111-148, §§ 1501(b), 10106(b), 124 Stat. 244, 909, as amended by Pub. L. No. 111-152, § 1002, 124 Stat. 1032. Exceptions may be available for certain individuals, such as those who cannot afford coverage or have been determined to have suffered hardships, members of Indian tribes, and those who qualify for religious reasons.

[38] Individuals who are eligible for Medicaid, Medicare, or other minimum essential coverage may purchase a policy through a PPACA exchange but will not be eligible for coverage subsidized by the PPACA premium tax credits, regardless of their household income.

[39] Household income is defined as the sum of a tax filer's modified adjusted gross income (i.e., adjusted gross income increased by amounts from tax-exempt interest, foreign earned income, and untaxed social security benefits) and the aggregate modified adjusted gross income of all other individuals for whom the tax filer is allowed a deduction for a personal exemption and who are required to file their own income tax returns for that taxable year.

[40] In determining Medicaid income eligibility, PPACA requires an income equivalent to 5 percent of the FPL to be disregarded from an individual's income. Therefore, the threshold for Medicaid eligibility will effectively increase from 133 percent of the FPL to 138 percent of the FPL in states that expand Medicaid. Accordingly, we refer to the Medicaid upper income threshold as up to 138 percent of the FPL. From 2014 through 2016, the federal government will pay 100 percent of the cost of providing coverage to individuals who are newly eligible for Medicaid in the states that opt to expand Medicaid. Starting in 2017, the federal government will gradually reduce its share each year until 2020 when it reaches 90 percent, which is the percentage it will pay thereafter.

[41] Individuals' eligibility for Medicaid depends on their states' current Medicaid eligibility standards. According to a recent report by the Kaiser Family Foundation, Medicaid eligibility for adults, including parents, is very limited in most states. The report found that in 17 states, the eligibility level for parents is below 50 percent of the FPL and nondisabled childless adults are typically not eligible for Medicaid regardless of their income level. See Kaiser Commission on Medicaid and the Uninsured. *How Will the Medicaid Expansion for Adults Impact Eligibility and Coverage* (Washington, D.C.: Kaiser Family Foundation, July 2012).

[42] If an individual chooses a more expensive plan than the reference plan (the secondlowest-cost-silver plan), the PPACA premium tax credit will not change and the individual will be responsible for the additional premium amount. If he or she chooses a plan with a less expensive premium than the reference plan, the individual will still be eligible to receive a PPACA premium tax credit up to the amount calculated based on the premium for the reference plan, which would reduce the amount of premium expenses the individual would have to pay.

[43] *See* Pub. L. No. 111-148, § 1402, 124 Stat.220, as amended by Pub. L. No. 111-152, § 1001(b), 124 Stat. 1031.

[44] If these maximum out-of-pocket limits had been in place in 2010 they would have been $5,950 for an individual and $11,900 for a family. These out-of-pocket limits are updated annually, so when these limits become effective in 2014 they will likely be different than what they would have been in 2010.

[45] Qualified individuals include U.S. citizens and lawful residents who are not incarcerated.

[46] Small Business Health Options Program exchanges, which are separate from the exchanges offering qualified health plans to individuals, are designed to help small businesses with up to 100 employees obtain a plan offered in the small group market in the state for their

employees. States may also elect to provide only one exchange for both qualified individuals and small employers if the exchange has adequate resources. Our study focuses on exchanges that will offer health insurance options in the individual market.

[47] HHS will establish and operate exchanges within states not electing to establish an exchange or that will not have an exchange operational by January 1, 2014. Pub. L. No. 111-148, § 1321(c), 124 Stat. 186. HHS will consider an exchange fully operational if it is capable of beginning operations by October 1, 2013 to support the initial open enrollment period.

[48] *See* 77 Fed. Reg. 70644, 70669 (to be codified at 45 C.F.R. Part 156, Subpart B).

[49] HHS has proposed a *de minimis variation* of +/-2 percentage points for the actuarial value associated with each metal tier (e.g., silver plans will be able to have actuarial values that range from 68 to 72 percent). *See* 77 Fed. Reg. 70644, 70671 (to be codified at 45 C.F.R. § 156.140). CCIIO officials told us, that in 2014, plans with actuarial values that do not fall within +/- 2 percentage points of one of the metal tiers will not be allowed to be sold either inside or outside of the PPACA exchanges.

[50] This assumes that HCTC participants with household incomes from 100 percent of the FPL to 400 percent of the FPL will likely be eligible for a PPACA premium tax credit.

[51] Household incomes at 100 percent of the FPL in 2010 ranged from $10,830 for an individual to $22,050 for a family of four in the 48 contiguous states and the District of Columbia.

[52] Household incomes at 400 percent of the FPL in 2010 ranged from $43,320 for an individual to $88,200 for a family of four in the 48 contiguous states and the District of Columbia.

[53] In 2012, the Congressional Budget Office and staff from the Joint Committee on Taxation reported that there is uncertainty about the future growth rate of private insurance premiums as a result of the insurance coverage provisions in PPACA. See Congressional Budget Office, *Estimates of the Effects of the Affordable Care Act on the Number of People Obtaining Employment-Based Health Insurance* (Washington, D.C.: March 2012). However, according to Congressional Budget Office projections, premiums for private health insurance per enrollee will increase by 5.7 percent per year, on average, between 2012 and 2022. See Congressional Budget Office, *Updated Estimates for the Insurance Coverage Provisions of the Affordable Care Act* (Washington, D.C.: March 2012). Another study from the Commonwealth Fund said that that the provisions in PPACA may help slow the rate of premium growth over time with a larger risk pool of younger, healthier people. See The Commonwealth Fund, *Help on the Horizon: How the Recession Has Left Millions of Workers Without Health Insurance, and How Health Reform Will Bring Relief* (Washington, D.C.: March 2011).

[54] We excluded all nonparticipants who were age 65 or older in 2010, and those for whom we were unable to obtain tax data. As a result, 390,203 of the 469,168 HCTC nonparticipants in 2010 were included in our analyses.

[55] For example, individuals who have access to employer-sponsored health plans may not be eligible for the PPACA premium tax credits.

[56] Department of Labor, *Selected Medical Benefits*. The report used data that the Department of Labor obtained from 2009 health plan documents as well as published survey data from the 2008 and 2009 Bureau of Labor Statistics National Compensation Survey (NCS), which were the most recently available NCS service-level data for health plans sponsored by private sector employers.

[57] *See* 77 Fed. Reg. 70644, 70649 (preamble to proposed rules, II. C. 2. c.). It is unknown whether the specific COBRA plans that HCTC participants are enrolled in cover these services, as the data sources that we reviewed on employer-sponsored health plans did not address these services.

[58] For any EHB category where a potential exchange benchmark plan lacks coverage, the plan will be supplemented to ensure that the plan covers services in all 10 EHB categories. For example, to ensure that plans cover habilitative services, HHS has proposed that plans either offer habilitative services at parity with rehabilitative services or determine which habilitative services they will cover and report those to HHS. *See* 77 Fed. Reg. 70644, 70670 (to be codified at 45 C.F.R. 156.115(a)(4).

[59] Department of Health and Human Services, Office of the Assistant Secretary for Planning and Evaluation, *Essential Health Benefits*.

[60] Department of Health and Human Services, Office of the Assistant Secretary for Planning and Evaluation, *Actuarial Value and Employer-Sponsored Insurance*.

[61] Jon R. Gabel et al., "More Than Half of Individual Health Plans Offer Coverage That Falls Short Of What Can Be Sold Through Exchanges As of 2014."

[62] Most of the plan officials we interviewed told us that the methods they used to calculate the actuarial values of the selected HCTC plans align with the February 2012 CCIIO *Actuarial Value and Cost-Sharing Reductions Bulletin*. However, for one of the selected HCTC plans, its actuarial value reflects the costs and utilization of a high-risk population and uses data reflective of that population in 2010 rather than of the plan's 2012 population.

[63] Jon R. Gabel et al., "More Than Half of Individual Health Plans Offer Coverage That Falls Short Of What Can Be Sold Through Exchanges As of 2014."

[64] This study used 2010 data on individual market plans from a sample of five states. We found that at least a third of the HCTC monthly participants enrolled in individual market plans in 2011 were from the five states that were sampled for the study.

[65] A change in the level of coverage, in general, will not affect the services that are covered as all plans in a given exchange will cover services on the basis of their exchange's EHB benchmark plan.

[66] While it is unknown how premium amounts may change in 2014, there will be restrictions under PPACA on the extent to which health insurance issuers who offer coverage through the exchanges can vary premiums. For example, health insurance issuers will still be able to vary premiums to a certain extent on the basis of age, tobacco use, family size, and geography, but they will no longer be allowed to vary premiums on the basis of factors such as health status, gender, or preexisting conditions.

[67] In addition, other PPACA provisions requiring changes across the health insurance market are already affecting or will soon affect health plans, including many HCTCqualified plans and plans that will be purchased through the PPACA exchanges. For example, lifetime limits that plans placed on essential benefits were prohibited in all individual market and group plans for plan years starting on or after September 23, 2010, and annual limits that plans placed on essential benefits are gradually being phased out for most health plans and will be prohibited by 2014. Pub. L. No. 111-148, §§ 1001(5), 10101(a), 124 Stat. 130, 883.

[68] Participants who are exempt from the tax penalty will have the option to purchase individual market catastrophic health plans through the PPACA exchanges that will have an actuarial value below 60 percent because these plans will be available to individuals who are exempt from the tax penalty (and available to individuals under the age of 30). However, even though these participants will have the option to purchase this coverage, it is unlikely that they will because the cost of their premium will be high relative to their income and the lower actuarial value of the plans will increase the potential costs of accessing covered services.

In: Health Care in the United States
Editor: Leone Giangiulio
ISBN: 978-1-62618-413-8

Chapter 4

PERSONAL CARE SERVICES: TRENDS, VULNERABILITIES, AND RECOMMENDATIONS FOR IMPROVEMENT*

U.S. Department of Health and Human Services, Office of Inspector General

EXECUTIVE SUMMARY

The Office of Inspector General's (OIG) body of work examining Medicaid personal care services (PCS) has found significant and persistent compliance, payment, and fraud vulnerabilities that demonstrate the need for Centers for Medicare & Medicaid Services (CMS) to take a more active role with States to combat these issues.

In 2011, Medicaid costs for PCS totaled approximately $12.7 billion, a 35-percent increase since 2005. Several Federal court decisions and Department of Health and Human Services policy initiatives aimed at providing more home and community-based options to Medicaid beneficiaries contribute to the increase in PCS use. As more and more State Medicaid programs explore home care options like PCS, it is critical that adequate safeguards exist to

* This is an edited, reformatted and augmented version of a U.S. Department of Health and Human Services, Office of Inspector General publication, dated November 2012.

prevent fraud, waste, and abuse in PCS and other important home care benefits.

This document summarizes OIG's PCS work and, on the basis of the analysis of this work in the aggregate, offers recommendations to improve the integrity of Medicaid PCS.

SUMMARY OBSERVATIONS

Improper Payments Linked to Lack of Compliance. As of August 2012, OIG has produced 23 audit and evaluation reports since 2006 focusing on PCS. Although the objectives, methodologies, and scopes of these audits and evaluations differed, in many instances OIG found that PCS payments were improper because the services:

- were not provided in compliance with State requirements, were unsupported by documentation indicating they had been rendered,
- were provided during periods in which the beneficiaries were in institutional stays reimbursed by Medicare or Medicaid, and/or
- were provided by PCS attendants who did not meet State qualification requirements.

Inadequate Controls To Ensure Appropriate Payment and Quality of Care. OIG work has demonstrated that existing program safeguards intended to ensure medical necessity, patient safety, and quality and prevent improper payments were often ineffective. In one or more audits or evaluations, OIG found:

- inadequate controls in the prior authorization processes (i.e., the processes to determine whether the beneficiaries qualify for PCS services before they are rendered);
- lack of prepayment controls (e.g., electronic edits to deny claims for PCS services that overlap with institutional stays);
- inconsistent standards for, and monitoring of, the qualifications of PCS attendants; and
- problematic billing practices (e.g., claims that lack details regarding dates of service and/or the identity of the PCS attendants providing services).

PCS Fraud Is a Growing Concern. OIG's Office of Investigations and many State Medicaid Fraud Control Units report that the increasing volume of fraud involving PCS has become a top concern. The most commonly reported schemes involve conspiracies between PCS attendants and Medicaid beneficiaries to submit claims for services that either were never provided or were not allowed under program rules. Investigators have noted that self-directed Medicaid service models (i.e., those in which beneficiaries have decisionmaking authority over certain services and take direct responsibility for managing their services with the system of available supports), especially those that allow beneficiaries significant control over the selection and payment of PCS attendants, are particularly vulnerable to these fraud schemes.[1]

RECOMMENDATIONS TO IMPROVE PROGRAM INTEGRITY

On the basis of the body of OIG's PCS work, we recommend that CMS take the following actions:

1. More fully and effectively use authorities available under section 1102 and Title XIX of the Social Security Act to improve regulatory oversight and monitoring of Medicaid PCS programs. Toward that end, CMS should promulgate regulations to:
   a) Reduce significant variation in State PCS attendant qualification standards and the potential for beneficiary exposure to unqualified PCS attendants by establishing minimum Federal qualification standards applicable to all PCS reimbursed by Medicaid.
   b) Improve CMS's and States' ability to monitor billing and care quality by requiring States to (1) either enroll all PCS attendants as providers <u>or</u> require all PCS attendants to register with their State Medicaid agencies and assign each attendant a unique identifier and (2) require that PCS claims include the specific date(s) when services were performed and the identity of the rendering PCS attendants.
   c) Reduce significant variation in States' PCS laws and regulations by creating or expanding Federal requirements and issuing operational guidance for claims documentation, beneficiary assessments, plans of care, and supervision of attendants.

2. Issue guidance to States regarding adequate prepayment controls. For example, CMS should identify a list of needed controls, including the necessary claims edits to prevent inappropriate PCS payments during periods when beneficiaries are receiving institutional care. CMS should also offer design instructions to better ensure the operability of prepayment controls.
3. Consider whether additional controls are needed to ensure that PCS are allowed under program rules and are provided.
4. Take action to provide States with data suitable for identifying overpayments for PCS claims during periods when beneficiaries are receiving institutional care paid for by Medicare or Medicaid. While we understand that CMS makes Medicare data available to States, more could be done to ensure that Medicare data are compatible with States' systems; that States have the capacity to store the data necessary to identify improper Medicaid payments;and that States may crosswalk Medicare and Medicaid data to identify potential instances of fraud, waste, and abuse.
5. Address recommendations contained in prior OIG reports that remain unimplemented. (See page 13 for a list of some prior recommendations related to PCS that remain unimplemented.)

BACKGROUND

Personal care services (PCS) provide assistance to the elderly, people with disabilities, and individuals with chronic or temporary conditions so that they can remain in their homes and communities. PCS are currently offered as either a State plan optional benefit or through various demonstrations and waivers[2] in all 50 States. (See Appendix A for related authorities.) States that provide PCS through State plans must comply with the general Medicaid program requirements outlined in section 1902 of the Social Security Act. States providing PCS through demonstration or waiver authorities must adhere to the terms of the application approved by CMS.

Recent data suggest rapid growth in PCS. In 2011, Medicaid costs for PCS totaled approximately $12.7 billion, a 35-percent increase since 2005. Additionally, the U.S. Department of Labor, Bureau of Employment Statistics, in its *Occupational Outlook Handbook, 2010-11 Edition*, projected that employment of personal and home health aides will grow by 46 percent by 2018, much faster than the average of 10 percent for all occupations.

A key factor in this increase was the United States Supreme Court decision in *Olmstead v. L.C.* 527 U.S. 581 (1999), which held that unjustified institutionalization of people with disabilities is a violation of the Americans With Disabilities Act. The Department of Health and Human Services has promoted States' efforts to provide Medicaid beneficiaries who are elderly or have disabilities with the choice of remaining in their homes and communities, as opposed to moving to nursing homes or other institutional care options. For example, the Patient Protection and Affordable Care Act (ACA) of 2010 removed barriers to providing home and community-based services by allowing additional State plan amendment options, increasing States' timeframes to elect and renew PCS as a care option, and streamlining processes for accessing home and community-based services. The ACA also provided additional funding for programs supporting home care goals, such as the Money Follows the Person demonstration and the Community First Choice Option programs.

Personal Care Services, A Primer

What are PCS? PCS consist of nonmedical services supporting activities of daily living, including bathing, dressing, light housework, money management, meal preparation, and transportation. PCS are provided to vulnerable care-dependent persons, typically those who are elderly or infirm and/or have disabilities.

Who provides PCS? Typically, an attendant provides PCS. In many States, PCS attendants work for personal care agencies, which are enrolled in the Medicaid program and bill for services on the attendants' behalf. Some States require attendants to register or enroll with the State, but most do not. States may define specific qualification requirements for attendants, such as minimum age, education, and health status.

What are coverage rules for PCS? Medicaid covers PCS for eligible individuals through Medicaid State plan options and/or through Medicaid waiver and demonstration authorities approved by CMS. (See Appendix A for a list of authorities.) Medicare does not provide reimbursement of PCS.

Under Federal law, PCS must be provided in a home or another location specified by the State and must follow a plan of care subject to approval and/or authorized by the State Medicaid agency.

Although there are no Federal requirements for PCS attendants, States are required to develop qualifications or requirements for attendants to ensure quality of care.

As of August 2012, the Office of Inspector General (OIG) has produced 23 audit and evaluation reports since 2006 on PCS, which consistently have found payment, compliance, and oversight vulnerabilities, as well as quality-of-care concerns. (See Appendix B for a list of related PCS audit and evaluation reports and Appendix C for a list of prior OIG recommendations related to PCS that remain unimplemented by CMS and States.) Federal investigators and State Medicaid Fraud Control Units (MFCUs) have also observed an increase in suspected PCS fraud. What follows are summary observations based on vulnerabilities detected in OIG audits, evaluations, and investigations, as well as recommendations for corrective actions based on the body of OIG's PCS work. OIG work referenced throughout this document was conducted in accordance with the professional standards applicable to audits, evaluations, and investigations.

SUMMARY OBSERVATIONS

Improper Payments Linked to Lack of Compliance with Documentation, Plans of Care, Medical Supervision, and Qualification Requirements

As of August 2012, OIG has completed seven statewide audits and one citywide audit of PCS payments. Another statewide audit is in progress. Since 2009, seven of the eight completed audits have identified over $582 million in questioned costs. Table 1 lists the error rates,[3] questioned costs, and set-aside costs[4] from each of the eight completed audits:

Table 1. Error Rates, Questioned Costs, and Set-Aside Costs for PCS in Seven States and One City

State Maryland[8]	Error Rate[5] (Percentage) 0%	Questioned Costs[6] $0	Set Aside Costs[7] $0
West Virginia[9]	1.00%	$19,830	$0
Nebraska[10]	2.31%	$168,652	$4,482,438
New Jersey [11]	40.35%	$145,405,192	$0
New York[12]	31.78%	$100,335,472	$15,325,689
New York City[13]	18.01%	$275,327,274	$0
North Carolina[14]	16.31%	$41,734,368	$0
Washington[15]	20.17%	$19,438,693	$30,323,597

The seven audits that found overpayments noted several types of deficiencies:

- Hours claimed in the billings were not supported by documentation.[16]
- PCS services failed to meet State assessment and/or prior authorization requirements.[17]
- PCS services did not meet State supervision requirements.[18]
- PCS attendants did not meet State qualification and/or training requirements.[19]
- Claims included periods during which beneficiaries received institutional care covered

These States often failed to provide oversight to prevent improper payments in several ways, including:

- insufficient resources to adequately monitor their PCS programs, especially once they began to experience substantial growth;21
- inadequate controls in the States' prior authorization processes (i.e., the processes to determine whether beneficiaries qualify for services before they are rendered);[22]
- ineffectiveness of accrediting organizations to which the States delegated authority to ensure compliance with applicable State regulations;[23]
- failure to conduct monitoring site visits of PCS agencies that employed attendants, leaving the role of oversight largely to
- beneficiaries;[24] and
- inadequate controls to prevent paying improper PCS claims, including instances when PCS were claimed while the beneficiaries received institutional care.[25]

Separately, a 2010 OIG evaluation examining PCS in 10 States over a 1-year period found that 18 percent of paid claims for Medicaid PCS in a universe totaling $724 million were inappropriate because the required qualifications for PCS attendants were undocumented.[26] The most often undocumented qualifications were age, education, and the results of background checks. Although the insufficient documentation may be an indicator that PCS attendants or agencies did not maintain or have ready access to documents containing this information, it could signal that the sampled PCS attendants did not meet State qualifications designed to ensure patient safety and high quality of care.

Interviews with Medicaid Beneficiaries Reveal Quality-of-Care Concerns

In interviews conducted in connection with two OIG audits of PCS in New York City and New York State, the majority of sampled Medicaid beneficiaries interviewed (40 of the 65 beneficiaries in New York City and 38 of the 55 in New York State) reported to OIG quality- of-care problems with their PCS attendants. The most serious allegations included physical abuse or threats of abuse, property theft, and patient abandonment. One beneficiary reported that an attendant abandoned her on two occasions – in the street and in the subway – because the attendant's shift had ended.

Without proper control and oversight mechanisms, unqualified attendants could expose beneficiaries to substandard quality of care and injury.

Inadequate Controls to Ensure Appropriate Payment and Quality of Care

Inadequate Controls To Prevent PCS Payments During Institutional Care. PCS are generally not eligible for Federal financial participation when provided to a beneficiary receiving services as an inpatient or a resident at a hospital, nursing home, or other institution.27 However, OIG work has documented many instances when PCS providers received payment during periods when the beneficiary purportedly received institutional care service.

An audit examining paid PCS claims over a 30-month period in Nebraska identified 464 instances in which PCS providers billed and were improperly paid for PCS during the beneficiaries' inpatient hospital stays.[28] A 2008 evaluation of PCS payments in the first quarter of 2006 found that the five States reviewed paid nearly $500,000 for PCS on dates when beneficiaries were institutionalized in Medicaid-funded facilities.[29] This review cited problems with the States' claims payment systems, including unsuccessful prepayment edits, which could have contributed to the estimated $11 million in potentially improper payments over the 3-month period.[30]

Numerous OIG and MFCU investigations have focused on potentially false PCS claims during periods of beneficiary institutionalization, resulting in convictions of PCS attendants and their employers.[31]

Qualification Safeguards. To be eligible for Federal financial ., PCS must be provided by a qualified individual.[32] Although no Federal requirements that specify qualifications for PCS .ants, States are required to specify qualifications or requirements for S attendants to ensure quality of care. A 2006 evaluation of State requirements for PCS attendants revealed 301 different sets of requirements nationwide.[33] The most common requirements were background checks; training; supervision; minimum age; health status (e.g., that the attendant test negative for tuberculosis); and education (e.g., attainment of a high school diploma). The report noted that the wide variation among States and within the same State may make it difficult to ensure compliance with requirements. Additionally, a 2010 evaluation of compliance with qualification requirements in 10 States found that PCS attendant qualifications were undocumented for 18 percent of Medicaid PCS claims.[34] Additional Federal regulations that set minimum qualifications could improve consistency among States and better ensure that beneficiaries receive PCS from qualified PCS attendants.

Billing Policies That Impair Program Integrity Efforts. OIG work on PCS has identified two distinct problems with State billing policies. First, PCS claims often do not specify the dates when the services were actually provided, and second, PCS claims do not identify the attendant that provided the service(s).

Dates of Services Not Identified on Claims. The 2008 evaluation revealed that the claims data in three of five States reviewed could not be used to accurately identify overlapping claims. These States allow PCS providers to submit claims through a process commonly referred to as "span billing." In general, span billing allows providers to submit one claim requesting payment for multiple instances of PCS provided over a range of dates (week or month), without specifying dates when the services were actually provided. The inability to identify service dates on claims presents a significant oversight challenge because the State cannot determine whether, for example, PCS overlap with dates when the beneficiaries received institutional care services.[35]

The problematic consequences of span billing were seen in an evaluation focusing on PCS claims for services in excess of 24 hours per day and between 16 and 24 hours per day.[36] This review examined PCS claims in 5 States and identified 871 paid claims in 4 States that were for services provided in excess of 24 hours per day to a single beneficiary. It also identified over 2,000 other paid claims that totaled or nearly totaled 24 hours per day, a volume of services that could raise program integrity concerns.

During ad hoc interviews with MFCU directors in two States that allow span billing, the directors reported that they have recommended to their Medicaid agencies that span billing be prohibited. These MFCU directors reported that span billing prevents their investigators from obtaining necessary evidence to pursue fraud cases against PCS attendants and agencies. In some PCS fraud cases, investigators rely on evidence that compares the dates of services listed on Medicaid claims to dates when the PCS attendants were engaged in conflicting activities (e.g., other job, travel). When specific dates of service are not included on claims, fraud investigations could be significantly hindered. Additional Federal regulations requiring that all States require the dates of services on claims would improve Federal and State program integrity efforts.

Fraud Example

Owner Of Pcs Agency Sentenced For Defrauding Medicaid Out Of More Than $650,000

As a result of a joint investigation by Federal and State officials, John Alemoh Momoh, owner and operator of Hopecare Service, Inc., was sentenced to 2 years of incarceration and ordered to pay $656,876 in restitution to Medicaid.

Between May 2007 and March 2008, Momoh submitted claims that inflated the number of PCS hours provided to Medicaid beneficiaries. Momoh also submitted false claims for services that were not rendered, were provided by an unqualified individual, and were not medically necessary.

PCS Attendants Not Identified on Claims. Most States do not require PCS attendants to register with the State Medicaid programs and therefore do not assign PCS attendants unique identifiers to be included on claims.[37] As a result, conducting attendant-specific data mining and analysis in such States is difficult. Further, in the absence of information identifying the attendants, States are challenged to implement edits that would prevent payments or trigger prepayment reviews of claims associated with high-risk or excluded PCS attendants.[38] Similarly, the absence of the identity of the attendant on PCS claims forms creates significant challenges to law enforcement efforts to investigate potentially fraudulent claims. For this reason, numerous MFCUs have recommended to their State Medicaid agencies that PCS attendants be assigned unique identifiers that would appear on claims forms.[39] If States registered or enrolled PCS attendants and required attendant identifiers on claims, State and Federal program integrity staff could search for and follow up on questionable billing patterns (e.g., billings for more than 24 hours in a day or for other impossible or improbable numbers of hours) and implement edits to prevent improper claims.

PCS Fraud Is a Growing Concern

OIG and the MFCUs have noted an increasing amount of fraud cases involving PCS. As of 2010, MFCUs had more open investigations involving PCS fraud than any other type of Medicaid service, with more than 1,000 investigations nationwide. In a recent survey, MFCUs cited fraud occurring in home and community-based settings, consisting mostly of PCS fraud, as a top fraud concern affecting their States.[40]

Cases investigated by OIG's Office of Investigations (OI) and discussions with multiple MFCUs indicate that the most common fraud schemes involve conspiracies between PCS attendants and beneficiaries. In a growing number of instances, the beneficiaries are being charged as coconspirators because they accepted cash or other benefits in exchange for participating in the fraud. These cases appear to be especially prevalent in States using CMS-approved home and community-based service waivers that allow relatives of beneficiaries to be their PCS attendants.[41] In many of these cases, investigation reveals that the beneficiaries do not appear to have the medical conditions or physical limitations documented on their assessments and therefore are not eligible for PCS.[42]

Additionally, OI and the MFCUs are encountering a new fraud scenario in States with self-directed Medicaid service models (i.e., those in which beneficiaries have decisionmaking authority over certain services and are directly responsible for managing their services with the system of available supports) and particularly in those States that send payment for PCS services directly to the beneficiaries instead of the attendants.[43] Although State Medicaid programs in these States require beneficiaries to give the payments to the PCS attendants, cases in which beneficiaries submit false claims for services that were never provided are now being prosecuted. In such cases, the beneficiaries typically forge the PCS attendants' names and then deposit the checks into their own bank accounts.[44] In States allowing self-directed PCS models, additional controls may be necessary to ensure that services both are necessary and are provided.

Fraud is often difficult to detect by reviewing documentation alone. The majority of the overpayments identified in OIG audits are the consequence of missing documentation that services were performed, assessments were conducted, training and qualification requirements were met, and plans of care were completed. In contrast, fraud is often proven by showing that the existing documentation of such activities by PCS attendants and providers is false (see the fraud example on the previous page).

At present, most fraud cases involving PCS come to the attention of law enforcement only through referrals from individuals who know the persons committing the acts. However, if the availability and quality of PCS data were improved, data could be analyzed to identify and follow up on aberrancies and questionable billing patterns. For example, PCS attendants and agencies that commit fraud often bill for impossibly or improbably large volumes of services; for services that conflict with one another (e.g., a PCS attendant purports to provide many hours of services to multiple beneficiaries on the same dates); or for services that could not have been performed as claimed because of geographical distances between beneficiaries purportedly served by the same PCS attendant on the same day. If claims contained more specific details, including the exact dates of service and the identity of the PCS attendants, such irregular billings could be more easily and systematically discovered through claims analysis by State program integrity units.

RECOMMENDATIONS TO IMPROVE PROGRAM INTEGRITY

On the basis of the body of OIG's PCS work, we recommend that CMS take the following actions:

1. More fully and effectively use authorities available under section 1102 and Title XIX of the Social Security Act to improve regulatory oversight and monitoring of Medicaid PCS programs. Toward that end, CMS should promulgate regulations to:
   a) Reduce significant variation in State PCS attendant qualification standards and the potential for beneficiary exposure to unqualified PCS attendants by establishing minimum Federal qualification standards applicable to all PCS reimbursed by Medicaid. For example, CMS could establish minimum age and education

standards and requirements for screening attendants (e.g., criminal background and Federal and State exclusion checks). These standards could be informed by work currently being conducted by the CMS-funded National Direct Service Workforce Resource Center (the Resource Center), which plans to develop a set of core competencies for workers providing long-term services. CMS could also consider the results of its National Background Check program, which has awarded selected States with funding to design a comprehensive national background check program for jobs involving direct patient care.

b) Improve CMS's and States' ability to monitor billing and care quality by requiring States to (1) either enroll all PCS attendants as providers or require all PCS attendants to register with their State Medicaid agencies and assign each attendant a unique identifier and (2) require that PCS claims include the specific date(s) when services were performed and the identity of the rendering PCS attendants.

c) Reduce significant variation in States' PCS laws and regulations by creating or expanding Federal requirements and issuing operational guidance for claims documentation, beneficiary assessments, plans of care, and supervision of attendants.

2. Issue guidance to States regarding adequate prepayment controls. For example, CMS should identify a list of needed controls, including the necessary claims edits to prevent inappropriate PCS payments during periods when beneficiaries are receiving institutional care. CMS should also offer design instructions to better ensure the operability of prepayment controls.
3. Consider whether additional controls are needed to ensure that PCS are allowed under program rules and are provided. For example, as part of its State Plan and waiver application process, CMS could require States to identify specific safeguards to prevent the fraud schemes highlighted in this report.
4. Take action to provide States with data suitable for identifying overpayments for PCS claims during periods when beneficiaries are receiving institutional care paid for by Medicare or Medicaid. While we understand that CMS makes Medicare data available to States, more could be done to ensure that Medicare data are compatible with States' systems; that States have the capacity to store the data necessary to identify improper Medicaid payments; and that States

may crosswalk Medicare and Medicaid data to identify potential instances of fraud, waste, and abuse.

5. Address recommendations contained in prior OIG reports that remain unimplemented. (See Appendix C for a list of some prior recommendations related to PCS that remain unimplemented.)

Agency Comments and Office of Inspector General Response

We made five recommendations in the report. CMS concurred with our fourth recommendation but did not indicate whether it concurred with our first, second, or third recommendations. Our fifth recommendation related to addressing prior unimplemented OIG recommendations. CMS indicated that it will incorporate those recommendations when developing action plans to address recommendations from this report. CMS generally agreed that more needs to be done at the Federal and State level to ensure appropriate billing for provided PCS.

More specifically, with regard to recommendation 1.a., CMS noted that in 2011 it funded the development of the *Road Map of Core Competencies for the Direct Service Workforce;* the direct service workforce will include PCS attendants. CMS expects this project to produce a set of service worker competencies by 2014, which CMS will then encourage States to adopt for use in their PCS programs. The agency also stated that it will continue to work with States on the National Background Check program.

We support CMS's work to develop core competencies that include minimum standards that any PCS attendant must have in order to be considered qualified to render PCS. However, on the basis of OIG's work documenting that States and local jurisdictions have developed over 300 PCS attendant requirements in the absence of Federal qualification requirements, we remain concerned that States will not adopt any core competencies unless CMS requires them to do so. For that reason and because of the overpayments for unqualified PCS attendants identified in prior work, we continue to recommend that CMS establish minimum Federal qualification standards applicable to all Medicaid-reimbursed PCS.

In relation to recommendation 1.b. (1), CMS stated that it will explore and identify the potential costs and benefits of States' either enrolling all PCS attendants as providers or requiring that attendants register with their State

Medicaid agencies. In addition, CMS indicated that it would explore and identify improvements to claims documentation that facilitate accurate payments and the detection of fraud and abuse. We reiterate that CMS's and States' ability to monitor billing and care quality could be improved by assigning PCS attendants unique identifiers through either an enrollment or registration process and by requiring these identifiers, as well as the specific dates of service, on claims. We continue to recommend that CMS promulgate related regulations.

In relation to recommendation 1.c., CMS outlined regulations that are part of the Community First Choice (CFC) benefit that the agency reported would standardize requirements for both care plans and assessments. CMS noted that the same requirements appear in its proposed regulations for home and community-based services provided under sections 1915(c) and 1915(i) of the Social Security Act. We appreciate that in new programs, such as CFC, CMS is working to address some of the issues we have raised in this report. We ask that in its final management decision, CMS provide further explanation as to how the regulations it referenced will serve to standardize States' care plans and assessments. We augmented our report to recommend that CMS issue guidance outlining expectations regarding how the regulations CMS referenced should be implemented to achieve standardization and improvements in claims documentation, beneficiary assessments, plans of care, and supervision of attendants.

In relation to our second recommendation, CMS stated that it intends to issue guidance to remind States of their obligation to review their own data to identify payment and utilization aberrations. CMS also stated that it will begin using its own data sources to better identify claims outliers, review those findings regularly with States, provide technical assistance to States on implementing those practices, share the findings of our report with States, and work with national long-term-care associations to improve program integrity in Medicaid PCS. We would appreciate CMS's providing a timetable for implementation of each of these activities in its final management decision.

In relation to our third recommendation, CMS stated that it plans to provide States with guidance on educating PCS providers on the program integrity issues identified in our report. CMS indicated it will also consult with stakeholders and attempt to create and publish guidance for States about program integrity controls through various technical assistance vehicles. We request that in its final management decision, CMS provide a timeline for development and completion of these activities. Furthermore, CMS identified several fraud protections it believes currently exist in its self-directed waiver service models. While we agree that the existing protections CMS described are important, they have not succeeded in preventing the vulnerabilities found in our reviews, audits, and investigations. We continue to recommend that CMS consider additional controls to ensure that PCS are allowed under program rules and are provided.

CMS concurred with our fourth recommendation and indicated that it will work with the Medicare and Medicaid Coordination Office to identify additional data-sharing approaches with States for dually eligible beneficiaries to prevent overpayments for PCS claims.

In response to our fifth recommendation, CMS stated that prior OIG recommendations that are contained in Appendix C appear to be largely encompassed within the first four recommendations in this report. CMS therefore said that it will incorporate its response to the prior recommendations as part of its actions to address our first through fourth recommendations. OIG continues to consider the prior recommendations as unimplemented and encourages CMS to take actions that address all recommendations in this report as well as our prior recommendations. OIG will consider whether specific actions taken by CMS address the PCS issues and recommendations identified in this report and the reports listed in Appendix C.

We ask that in its final management decision, CMS more clearly indicate whether it concurs with our recommendations 1(a)-(c), 2, 3, and 5.

Appendix A –Personal Care Services – Related Authorities Under Title XIX of the Social Security Act

States can provide personal care services (PCS) to eligible Medicaid beneficiaries through State plan and waiver programs. States that provide PCS through State plan programs must comply with the general Medicaid program requirements in section 1902 of the Social Security Act. States can also provide PCS through 1115 demonstration; 1915(a) and 1915(b) managed care and freedom of choice; 1915(c) home and community-based services waiver; 1915(j) self-directed personal assistant services; 1915(k) community first choice programs; and 1915(i), which allows PCS under a State amendment option.

APPENDIX B - LIST OF RELATED OIG REPORTS

Report	*Issue Date*
States' Requirements for Medicaid-Funded Personal Care Service Attendants (OEI-07-05-00250)	December 2006
Review of Personal Care Services Claimed by the Center for Living and Workings, Inc. (A-01-06-00011)	October 2007
Payments Made in Error for Personal Care Services During Institutional Stays (OEI-07-06-00620)	August 2008
Medicaid-Funded Personal Care Services in Excess of 24 Hours per Day (OEI-07-06-00621)	October 2008
Partnership Review of Medicaid Claims Processed by Cerebral Palsy and Stavros for Personal Care Attendant Services Provided to Beneficiaries during Inpatient Stays (A-01-08-00001)	November 2008
Review of Medicaid Personal Care Services Claims Made by Providers in New York City (A-02-07-01054)	June 2009
Review of Medicaid Personal Care Service Claims Submitted by Independence First, Inc. and Claimed by Wisconsin From July 1, 2006, Through June 30, 2008 (A-05-09-00093)	April 2010
Review of Medicaid Personal Care Service Claims Submitted by Dane County Department of Human Services and Claimed by Wisconsin From July 1, 2006, Through June 30, 2008 (A-05-10-00018)	September 2010
Review of Medicaid Personal Care Service Claims Submitted by Clarity Care, Inc., and Claimed by Wisconsin From July 1, 2006, Through June 30, 2008 (A-05-10-00019)	October 2010
Review of Medicaid Personal Care Services Claims Made by Providers in New York State (A-02-08-01005)	October 2010
Review of Personal Care Services Provided by Tri-State Home Health and Equipment Services, Inc., in the District of Columbia (A-03-08-00207)	November 2010

Inappropriate Claims for Medicaid Personal Care Services (OEI-07-08-00430)	December 2010
Review of Federal Reimbursement Claimed by North Carolina for Medicaid Personal Care Services Claims Submitted by Shipman Family Home Care, Inc. (A-04-09-04041)	February 2011
Review of New Mexico Medicaid Personal Care Services Provided by Ambercare Home Health (A-06-09-00062)	March 2011
Review of Medicaid Personal Care Services Claimed by Washington State (A-09-09-00030)	June 2011
Review of Medicaid Personal Care Services Claims Submitted by Providers in North Carolina (A-04-10-04003)	June 2011
Nebraska Medicaid Payments for Personal Care Services (A-07-10-03152)	July 2011
Review of Personal Care Services Claimed Under Maryland's Medicaid State Plan (A-03-11-00200)	November 2011
Review of Medicaid Personal Care Claims Submitted by Providers in New Jersey (A-02-09-01002)	December 2011
Review of New Mexico Medicaid Personal Care Services Provided by Heritage Home Healthcare (A-06-09-00063)	May 2012
Review of New Mexico Medicaid Personal Care Services Provided by Clovis Homecare, Inc. (A-06-09-00117)	June 2012
Review of Louisiana Medicaid Personal Care Services Provided by American Pride Caregivers, LLC (A-06-09-00107)	June 2012
West Virginia Complied With Certain Federal Requirements for Most of the Personal Care Services Claimed for Its Aged and Disabled Waiver Program (A-03-11-00205)	June 2012

APPENDIX C – LIST OF CERTAIN UNIMPLEMENTED RECOMMENDATIONS FOR PERSONAL CARE SERVICES*

Recommendations to CMS

1. Work with States to reduce erroneous Medicaid payments for personal care services (PCS) provided during institutional stays (Payments Made in Error for Personal Care Services During Institutional Stays, OEI-07-06-00620) (CMS concurred.)
2. Enforce existing Federal Medicaid payment policies prohibiting Medicaid reimbursement for PCS provided over a range of dates if the range includes dates on which the beneficiary was institutionalized (Payments Made in Error for Personal Care Services During Institutional Stays, OEI-07-06-00620) (CMS did not concur.)
3. Work with States to ensure that agencies and attendants are aware of attendant qualification and documentation requirements and that Medicaid claims for PCS provided by attendants with undocumented qualifications are not paid (Inappropriate Claims for Medicaid Personal Care Services, OEI 07-08-00430) (CMS concurred.)

Recommendations to Specific Medicaid State Agencies

1. Implement prepayment controls to monitor PCS claims for compliance with State requirements (Review of Personal Care Services Provided by Tri-State Home Health and Equipment Services, Inc., in the District of Columbia, A-03-08-00207) (The Department of Health Care Finance concurred.)
2. Provide more effective monitoring of PCS attendants' compliance with qualification requirements (Review of Personal Care Services Provided by Tri-State Home Health and Equipment Services, Inc., in the District of Columbia, A-03-08-00207) (The Department of Health Care Finance concurred.)
3. Strengthen controls by developing policies and procedures for more substantive documentation and prepayment and postpayment claim review to ensure that PCS claims are reviewed and paid in accordance with Federal and State requirements (Nebraska Medicaid Payments

for Personal Care Services, A-07-10-03152) (The Department of Health & Human Services concurred.)

*This list does not include overpayment recovery recommendations included in some OIG reports.

End Notes

[1] Additional information on self-directed Medicaid services is available at http://www.medicaid.gov/MedicaidCHIP-Program-Information/By-Topics/Delivery-Systems/Self-Directed-Services.html. Accessed on April 24, 2012.

[2] Section 1115 waivers give States flexibility to design and improve the Medicaid and Children's Health Insurance Program (CHIP) programs. Waivers let States test new or existing ways to deliver and pay for program coverage. The Centers for Medicare & Medicaid Services (CMS) conducts and sponsors a number of innovative demonstration projects to test and measure the effect of potential program changes. Additional information on section 1115 waivers and demonstrations is available at http://www.medicaid.gov/Medicaid-CHIP-Program-Information/ByTopics/Waivers/1115/Section-1115-Demonstration.html. Accessed on August 15, 2012.

[3] We calculated the error rate for each review by dividing the point estimate for the estimated value of unallowable items by the value of the sampling frame. These amounts can be found in the sampling methodology within the appendix of each report.

[4] The questioned costs and the set-aside costs are the lower limits of 90-percent confidence intervals. These amounts can be found in the sampling methodology within the appendix of each report.

[5] We calculated the error rate for each review by dividing the point estimate for the estimated value of unallowable items by the value of the sampling frame. These amounts can be found in the sampling methodology within the appendix of each report.

[6] "Questioned cost" means a cost that is questioned by OIG because of (1) an alleged violation of a provision of a law, regulation, contract, grant, cooperative agreement, or other agreement or document governing the expenditure of funds; (2) a finding that at the time of the audit, such cost is not supported by adequate documentation; or (3) a finding that the expenditure of funds for the intended purpose is unnecessary or unreasonable.

[7] Set-aside costs are generally costs that we believe are in error but the magnitude of which may not be statistically measurable or for which the criteria for determining the costs' propriety were not clearly set forth by the administering agency.

[8] Review of Personal Care Services Claimed Under Maryland's Medicaid State Plan (A-03-11-00200), November 2011.

[9] West Virginia Complied With Certain Federal Requirements for Most of the Personal Care Services Claimed for Its Aged and Disabled Waiver Program (A-03-11-00205), June 2012.

[10] Nebraska Medicaid Payments for Personal Care Services (A-07-10-03152), July 2011.

[11] Review of Personal Care Claims Submitted by Providers in New Jersey (A-02-09-01002), December 2011.

[12] Review of Medicaid Personal Care Services Claims Made by Providers in New York State (A-02-08-01005), October 2010.

[13] Review of Medicaid Personal Care Services Claims Made by Providers in New York City (A-02-07-01054), June 2009.

[14] Review of Medicaid Personal Care Services Claims Submitted by Providers in North Carolina (A-04-10-04003), June 2011.

[15] Review of Medicaid Personal Care Services Claimed by Washington State (A-09-09-00030), June 2011.

[16] Review of Medicaid Personal Care Services Claims Made by Providers in New York State (A-02-08-01005), October 2010; Review of Medicaid Personal Care Services Claimed by Washington State (A-09-09-00030), June 2011; Review of Medicaid Personal Care Services Claims Submitted by Providers in North Carolina (A-04-10 04003), June 2011; Nebraska Medicaid Payments for Personal Care Services (A-07-10-03152), July 2011; Review of Personal Care Claims Submitted by Providers in New Jersey (A-02-09-01002), December 2011; and West Virginia Complied With Certain Federal Requirements for Most of the Personal Care Services Claimed for Its Aged and Disabled Waiver Program (A-03-11-00205), June 2012.

[17] Review of Medicaid Personal Care Services Claims Made by Providers in New York State (A-02-08-01005), October 2010; Review of Medicaid Personal Care Services Claimed by Washington State (A-09-09-00030), June 2011; Review of Medicaid Personal Care Services Claims Submitted by Providers in North Carolina (A-04-10- 04003), June 2011; Nebraska Medicaid Payments for Personal Care Services (A-07-10-03152), July 2011; and Review of Personal Care Claims Submitted by Providers in New Jersey (A-02-09-01002), December 2011.

[18] Review of Medicaid Personal Care Services Claims Made by Providers in New York City (A-02-07-01054), June 2009; Review of Medicaid Personal Care Services Claims Made by Providers in New York State (A-02-08-01005), October 2010; Review of Medicaid Personal Care Services Claims Submitted by Providers in North Carolina (A-04- 10-04003), June 2011; and Review of Personal Care Claims Submitted by Providers in New Jersey (A-02-09- 01002), December 2011.

[19] Review of Medicaid Personal Care Services Claims Made by Providers in New York State (A-02-08-01005), October 2010; Review of Medicaid Personal Care Services Claimed by Washington State (A-09-09-00030), June 2011; Review of Medicaid Personal Care Services Claims Submitted by Providers in North Carolina (A-04-10- 04003), June 2011; and Review of Personal Care Claims Submitted by Providers in New Jersey (A-02-09-01002), December 2011.

[20] Nebraska Medicaid Payments for Personal Care Services (A-07-10-03152), July 2011.

[21] Review of Medicaid Personal Care Services Claims Submitted by Providers in North Carolina (A-04-10-04003), June 2011.

[22] Review of Personal Care Claims Submitted by Providers in New Jersey (A-02-09-01002), December 2011.

[23] Ibid.

[24] Nebraska Medicaid Payments for Personal Care Services (A-07-10-03152), July 2011. Failure to conduct onsite reviews of providers was also identified as a cause of payment of improper claims in New York State and New York City. Review of Medicaid Personal Care Services Claims Made by Providers in New York City (A-02-07-01054), June 2009, and Review of Medicaid Personal Care Services Claims Made by Providers in New York State (A-02-08- 01005), October 2010.

[25] Review of Medicaid Personal Care Services Claimed by Washington State (A-09-09-00030), June 2011; Nebraska Medicaid Payments for Personal Care Services (A-07-10-03152), July

2011; and West Virginia Complied With Certain Federal Requirements for Most of the Personal Care Services Claimed for Its Aged and Disabled Waiver Program (A-03-11-00205), June 2012.

[26] Inappropriate Claims for Medicaid Personal Care Services (OEI-07-08-00430), December 2010.

[27] For State Plan PCS, see Social Security Act § 1905(a)(24); 42 CFR § 440.167; regarding waivers, see 42 § 441.301(b)(1)(ii); 42 CFR § 440.70(c).

[28] Nebraska Medicaid Payments for Personal Care Services (A-07-10-03152), July 2011.

[29] Payments Made in Error for Personal Care Services During Institutional Stays (OEI-07-06-00620), August 2008.

[30] Ibid. The review also identified a large number of overpayments for PCS during dates when the beneficiaries were institutionalized in Medicare-paid facilities. The report recommended that CMS explore ways to ensure that State Medicaid programs have complete information on Medicare institutionalizations for dually eligible beneficiaries.

[31] A list of convictions may be found in OIG's compilation of "State Enforcement Actions." Available at https://oig.hhs.gov/fraud/enforcement/state/index.asp. Accessed on April 24, 2012.

[32] For State Plan PCS, see Social Security Act § 1905(a)(24); 42 CFR § 440.167; regarding waivers, see 42 CFR § 441.301(b)(1)(ii); 42 CFR § 440.70(c).

[33] States' Requirements for Medicaid-Funded Personal Care Service Attendants (OEI-07-05-00250), December 2006. The report noted that at the time of the review, there were 238 separate programs through which States were providing personal care services: 31 State plans and 207 Medicaid waivers.

[34] Inappropriate Claims for Medicaid Personal Care Services (OEI-07-08-00430), December 2010.

[35] For example, if a beneficiary was institutionalized from October 1 through October 7 and 10 hours of PCS were billed for the date range October 3 through October 9, the State cannot determine whether the PCS were provided between October 3 and October 6, when the beneficiary was institutionalized, or between October 7 and October 9, when the beneficiary was at home.

[36] Medicaid-Funded Personal Care Services in Excess of 24 Hours per Day (OEI-07-06-00621), October 2008.

[37] At least four States require enrollment of at least some of their Medicaid personal care attendants. Minnesota enrolls all attendants providing both State plan and waiver PCS, regardless of whether the attendants are self-employed or are employees of PCS agencies. Iowa enrolls all attendants providing waiver PCS. (Iowa does not have a State plan PCS benefit.) For both State plan and waiver PCS, Ohio enrolls all PCS attendants who are not employees of PCS agencies. Florida requires enrollment of attendants who are not employees of PCS agencies and are providing services under the State PCS plan.

[38] OIG's List of Excluded Individuals/Entities (LEIE) provides information to the health care industry, patients, and the public regarding individuals and entities currently excluded from participation in Medicare, Medicaid, and all other Federal health care programs. Individuals and entities who have been reinstated are removed from the LEIE. Additional information on excluded providers is available at https://oig.hhs.gov/faqs/exclusions-faq.asp. Accessed on August 15, 2012.

[39] MFCUs in Ohio, Washington, New Mexico, and Louisiana have notified OIG that they have made such recommendations.

[40] Based on MFCU responses to the survey conducted through the US DHHS-OIG Public-Private information Sharing Project, released through a Freedom of Information Act request in September 2011.

[41] Section 1915(c) Home and Community-Based Services waivers authorize States to provide long-term care in home and community-based settings rather than institutional settings. Additional information on these waivers is available at http://www.medicaid.gov/Medicaid-CHIP-Program-Information/ByTopics/Waivers/Waivers.html?filterBy=1915(c)#waivers. Accessed on June 20, 2012.

[42] Based on interviews with State officials and recommendations submitted to States by MFCUs in Missouri, Louisiana, Ohio, and Washington.

[43] Additional information on self-directed Medicaid services is available at http://www.medicaid.gov/MedicaidCHIP-Program-Information/By-Topics/Delivery-Systems/Self-Directed-Services.html. Accessed on April 24, 2012.

[44] An example of beneficiary submission of false claims for PCS is described in, "West Springfield Woman Pleads Guilty, Sentenced in Connection with Stealing Over $130,000 from Medicaid," May 3, 2011. Available at http://www.mass.gov/ago/news-and-updates/press-releases/2011/woman-pleads-guilty-sentenced-stealing130000.html. Accessed on April 24, 2012.

In: Health Care in the United States
Editor: Leone Giangiulio

ISBN: 978-1-62618-413-8

Chapter 5

TRADITIONAL VERSUS BENCHMARK BENEFITS UNDER MEDICAID*

Elicia J. Herz

SUMMARY

The Medicaid program, which served 69 million people in FY2011, finances the delivery of a wide variety of preventive, primary and acute care services as well as long-term services and supports for certain low-income populations. Benefits are available to beneficiaries through two avenues. First, the traditional Medicaid program covers a wide variety of mandatory services (e.g., inpatient hospital services, lab/x-ray services, physician care, nursing facility care for persons aged 21 and over) and other services at state option (e.g., prescribed drugs, physician-directed clinic services, physical therapy, prosthetic devices) to the majority of Medicaid beneficiaries across the United States. Within broad federal guidelines, states define the amount, duration, and scope of these benefits. Thus, even mandatory services are not identical from stateto-state.

The Deficit Reduction Act of 2005 (DRA; P.L. 109-171) created an alternative benefit structure for Medicaid. Under this authority, states may enroll certain Medicaid subpopulations into benchmark benefit plans that include four choices: (1) the standard Blue Cross/Blue Shield preferred provider plan under the Federal Employees Health Benefits

* This is an edited, reformatted and augmented version of a Congressional Research Service publication, CRS Report for Congress R42478, prepared for Members and Committees of Congress, from www.crs.gov, dated August 3, 2012.

Program, (2) a plan offered to state employees, (3) the largest commercial health maintenance organization in the state, and (4) other coverage appropriate for the targeted population, subject to approval by the Secretary of Health and Human Services (HHS).

Since the enactment of the Patient Protection and Affordable Care Act in 2010 (ACA; P.L. 111- 148, as amended), benchmark benefits have taken on a new importance in the Medicaid program. As per the ACA, a new mandatory group of non-elderly, non-pregnant adults with income up to 133% of the federal poverty level will be eligible for Medicaid beginning in 2014, or sooner at state option. These individuals will be required to enroll in benchmark plans rather than traditional Medicaid (with some exceptions for subgroups with special medical needs). However, to date, only a handful of states have experience administering these plans, nearly all of which have been tailored to specific subpopulations.

The Congressional Budget Office (CBO) and the Joint Committee on Taxation (JCT) estimated that coverage expansion provisions in the ACA would increase enrollment by about 7 million in FY2014, rising to 11 million by FY2022 in both the Medicaid and the State Children's Health Insurance Programs (Congressional Budget Office, Estimates for the Insurance Coverage Provisions of the Affordable Care Act Updated for the Recent Supreme Court Decision, July 2012). Many of these new enrollees will get benchmark benefits. To assist Congress in evaluating the current scope of benefits available under Medicaid, this report outlines the major rules that govern and define both traditional Medicaid and benchmark benefits. It also compares the similarities and differences between these two benefit package designs.

INTRODUCTION

Medicaid was established in 1965 to provide basic medical services to certain low-income populations. It is a means-tested entitlement program that financed the delivery of primary and acute medical services, as well as long-term services and supports, to more than an estimated 69 million people in FY2011.[1] The estimated annual cost to the federal and state governments for Medicaid was nearly $404 billion in FY2010.[2]

Each state designs and administers its own version of Medicaid under broad federal rules. State variability is the rule rather than the exception in terms of eligibility levels, covered services, and how those services are delivered and reimbursed.

Not everyone enrolled in Medicaid has access to the same set of services. Different eligibility classifications determine available benefits, as described below. This report begins with a summary of major Medicaid eligibility pathways. Then traditional Medicaid benefits and benchmark coverage are described.

The final section provides an analysis of state experiences with benchmark benefit packages as of early 2011. Additional CRS resources on the Medicaid and Children's Health Insurance Program are provided at the end of this report.

MEDICAID ELIGIBILITY

Historically, eligibility for Medicaid was subject to "categorical restrictions" that generally limited coverage to the elderly, persons with disabilities, members of families with dependent children, certain other pregnant women and children, among others. Recent changes in federal law established Medicaid eligibility for poor non-elderly, childless adults who do not fit into these traditional categories; states may cover such individuals now, but coverage of this new group will become mandatory beginning in 2014.

In addition, to qualify for Medicaid, applicants must have income (and sometimes assets) that meet financial requirements. These financial criteria are typically tied to certain federal cash assistance program rules or to specific percentages of the federal poverty level (FPL).[3]

Below is a description of services available for Medicaid beneficiaries by eligibility classification.

First, "categorical needy" individuals represent the vast majority of people enrolled in Medicaid, most of whom receive traditional Medicaid benefits (described in more detail below). The Patient Protection and Affordable Care Act (ACA; P.L. 111-148, as amended) requires that a newly established categorically needy group consisting of poor nonelderly, nonpregnant adults with income below 133% FPL receive Medicaid benchmark benefits, an alternative to traditional Medicaid benefits. However, on June 28, 2012, the United States Supreme Court issued a decision in *National Federation of Independent Business v. Sebelius*. The Court held that the federal government cannot terminate current Medicaid federal matching funds if a state refuses to expand its Medicaid program to include non-elderly, non-pregnant adults under 133% of the federal poverty level. If a state accepts the new ACA Medicaid expansion funds, it must abide by the new expansion coverage rules, but based on the Court's opinion, it appears that a state can refuse to participate in the expansion without losing any of its current Medicaid matching funds.[4]

Other benefit rules apply to individuals classified as "medically needy," including people who meet the main categorical restrictions described above but may have higher income.

States electing the medically needy option must provide coverage to certain pregnant women and children under age 18. For the medically needy, states may offer a more restrictive benefit package than is available to most categorically needy individuals.

Finally, states also use the authority in Section 1115 of the Social Security Act to tailor benefits to state-specified subpopulations that can include both currently authorized groups and/or new groups not specified in federal statute. Each such waiver delineates the unique terms and conditions that are negotiated between a given state and the federal Centers for Medicare & Medicaid Services (CMS).[5]

Table 1 provides examples of Medicaid benefits available by selected eligibility classifications. As illustrated, different Medicaid subpopulations may have access to benefit packages that can be quite varied. Additional details are described further below.

Traditional Medicaid Benefits

Like eligibility, under traditional Medicaid, states must cover certain benefits, while other services may be offered at state option. Examples of benefits that are mandatory for most Medicaid groups (i.e., categorically needy populations) include inpatient hospital services, physician services, laboratory and x-ray services, early and periodic screening, diagnostic and treatment services (EPSDT) for individuals under 21,[6] nursing facility services for individuals aged 21 and over, and home health care for those entitled to nursing facility care. Examples of optional benefits for such Medicaid groups include prescribed drugs, physician-directed clinic services, services of other licensed practitioners (e.g., chiropractors, podiatrists, psychologists) services, nursing facility services for individuals under age 21, physical therapy, and prosthetic devices.

Table 2 provides additional information for selected optional benefits covered by most states under the traditional Medicaid program.

Table 1. Examples of Medicaid Benefits by Eligibility Classification

Type of Benefit and Benefit Package		Eligibility Classification		
Type of Benefit	Categorically Needy	Medically Needy	Section 1115	Non-Elderly, Non-
	(excluding Non-Elderly, Non-Pregnant Adults)		Waivers	Pregnant Adults
Mandatory	-Inpatient hospital	-Prenatal and	-Negotiated between	-Benchmark plans
	-Nursing facility care (age 21+) - EPSDT (< age 21)	delivery services - Ambulatory services (< age 18; persons entitled to	the states and the Secretary of Health and Human Services (HHS)	
	-Physicians	institutional care)		
	-Federally-qualified	-Home health for		
	health centers	those entitled to		
	-Family planning	nursing facility care		
	-Pregnancy-related services			
Optional	-Clinic services	-Nursing facility care	-Negotiated between	-For special needs
	-Prescribed drugs	-Clinic services	the states and	subgroups, option to
	-Physical, occupational, and speech therapy - Other practitioners	-Physical, occupational, and speech therapy -Other practitioners	Secretary of HHS	have same benefits as categorically needy or enroll in benchmark plan
	-Dental	-Dental		
Traditional Benefits Versus Benchmark Package	Traditional Benefits	Traditional Benefits	Not applicable	Benchmark plans with exceptions; see Table 3 for details

Sources: Title XIX of the Social Security Act and related federal guidance.

Note: With respect to medically needy groups, broader requirements apply if a state has chosen to provide coverage for medically needy individuals in intermediate care facilities for the mentally retarded or in institutions for mental diseases. In these cases, states are required to cover either the same services as those which are mandatory for the categorically needy, or alternatively, the care and services described in seven of the first twenty-four paragraphs in the federal Medicaid statute defining covered mandatory and optional services. EPSDT means "early and periodic screening, diagnostic and treatment." This benefit includes well-child visits, immunizations, lab tests, as well as vision, dental and hearing screening services at regular intervals.

Table 2. Examples of Frequently Covered Optional Benefits Under Traditional Medicaid as of August 13, 2010

Selected Optional Benefits	Number of States Offering Benefit	Description of Benefit
	Examples of Preventive, Primary and Acute Care Services	
Clinic Services	50	A wide range of health care services including services for prevention or treatment of health conditions or illnesses, surgery, and other care provided in a centralized facility
Hospice Services	48	Care for persons with illnesses that cannot be cured or fully treated. Hospice care involves a team of medical professionals who take care of the medical, physical, social, emotional and spiritual needs of the patient, and also support to the patient's family or caregiver
Occupational Therapy	50	Services to enhance an individual's participation in, or performance of, common activities such as eating, dressing, moving about, working, and going to school
Optometric Services	50	Services from an individual with training to diagnose and prescribe treatment for diseases of the eye and problems with vision, and may include eye glasses, lenses, exercises or referrals for specialized treatment
Physical Therapy	50	Services to restore physical function to a person with a disability caused by illness, trauma, or birth defects
Prescribed Drugs	50	Drugs that an individual can get only if a doctor (or another authorized health care provider) gives permission through a prescription
Speech and Language Therapy	49	Services to diagnose and treat speech and language problems

Selected Optional Benefits	Number of States Offering Benefit	Description of Benefit
Targeted Case Management	50	Services to help individuals be independent and learn to manage their health care, including linking such people with health care providers, social services, educational services, etc., based on that person's needs
	Examples of Long-Term Services and Supports	
Inpatient Psychiatric Services for Individuals < Age 21	48	Services that a person < age 21 might receive at a hospital or psychiatric residential treatment facility while staying overnight for treatment of mental illness, and may include services provided by a physician or nurse, lab work, surgery, and drugs
Intermediate Care Facilities for the Mentally Retarded	51	Services at a facility that provides 24-hour rehabilitative as well as health care and services for persons with developmental disabilities
Nursing Facility Services for Individuals < Age 21	50	Skilled nursing, rehabilitation, and other services provided in a facility to assist individuals with illness, injuries, or other disabilities to recover or improve, and to provide long-term care to those who need support with daily activities such as bathing, dressing and eating
Prosthetic Devices	49	Devices to replace, correct or support missing or impaired portions of the body
Targeted Case Management for Mental Health	51	Services to help individuals with mental health needs learn how to manage their health care

Source: Centers for Medicare & Medicaid Services, derived from www.healthcare.gov and individual state Medicaid websites as of August 13, 2010, personal communication, fall of 2010.

Note: The definition of state includes the District of Columbia.

The breadth of coverage for a given benefit can and does vary from state to state, even for mandatory benefits. In general, in defining a covered benefit, federal guidelines require that (1) services be sufficient in amount, duration and scope to reasonably achieve their purpose; (2) the amount, duration, and scope of services must be the same statewide; and (3) with some exceptions, beneficiaries must have freedom of choice of providers among health care practitioners or managed care entities participating in Medicaid. States can modify these rules via existing waiver authority provided in Section 1115 of the Social Security Act.

Medicaid Benchmark Benefit Packages

As an alternative to providing all the mandatory and selected optional benefits under traditional Medicaid, the Deficit Reduction Act of 2005 (DRA; P.L. 109-171) gave states the option to enroll state-specified groups in benchmark and benchmark-equivalent benefit packages.[7] These plans can exist in sub-state areas and can be limited to specific subpopulations.

States can require "full benefit eligibles" (or specific subgroups of these individuals) to enroll in Medicaid benchmark benefits. A full benefit eligible is someone who is eligible for all the mandatory and optional services that a state covers under its traditional Medicaid program. Medically needy and certain spend-down populations (e.g., individuals whose Medicaid eligibility is based on a reduction of countable income for costs incurred for medical or remedial care) are excluded from the definition of a full benefit eligible. Specific groups are exempt from mandatory enrollment in benchmark benefit packages (e.g., those with special health care needs such as disabling mental disorders or serious and complex medical conditions). *Table 3* provides a description of each of these exempted populations.

Table 3. Statutory and Regulatory Exceptions to Mandatory Enrollment in Medicaid Benchmark Benefit Plans

(i) mandatory pregnant women with income below 133% of the federal poverty level (FPL)

(ii) blind or disabled individuals without regard to whether the individual is eligible for Supplemental Security Income (SSI) benefits and certain children under age 19 who meet the SSI disability definition, require an institutional level of care and the expected cost of care outside an appropriate institution is less than the expected cost that would be incurred within an appropriate institution; this latter group is sometimes referred to as the Katie Beckett group

(iii) Medicaid beneficiaries entitled to benefits under Medicare

(iv) terminally ill individuals receiving Medicaid hospice benefits

(v) inpatients in an institution who are required to pay for the costs of such care, excluding a minimal amount required for personal needs (e.g., hair care, clothing, telephone services)

(vi) certain persons who are medically frail or have special needs such as children under age 19 eligible for SSI, or foster care or other out-of-home placement, or those receiving foster care or adoption assistance, or receiving community-based services through certain Title V Maternal and Child Health grants

(vii) beneficiaries qualifying for long-term care services (e.g., nursing facility services or similar level of care in any institution, certain home and community-based waiver services (under Section 1915(c) and (d), and other optional state plan long-term care services)

(i) mandatory pregnant women with income below 133% of the federal poverty level (FPL)
certain children in foster care receiving child welfare services (under Title IV-B) or certain children for whom adoption or foster care assistance is made available (under Title IV-E), without regard to age

(viii) Temporary Assistance for Needy Families (TANF) and Section 1931(i) parents

(ix) optional breast and cervical cancer women (under age 65, with income below 250% FPL who are identified through the Centers for Disease Control screening program who need treatment for either of these cancers and are not eligible for other creditable coverage)

(x) limited services beneficiaries, including optional tuberculosis-infected individuals with income up to the level applicable to mandatory SSI populations, or individuals who are not a qualified alien (e.g., certain aliens lawfully admitted for permanent residence in the U.S.) and for whom only treatment of emergency medical conditions is covered (as per Section 1903(v))

Source: Section 1937(a)(2)(B) of the Social Security Act and 42 CFR 440.315.

These exempted groups may get traditional Medicaid benefits or may be offered voluntary enrollment in benchmark benefit plans. In such cases, states must describe the differences between traditional Medicaid and benchmark plans to these beneficiaries in order to facilitate an informed choice.

In general, benchmark benefit packages may cover fewer benefits than traditional Medicaid, but there are some requirements, such as coverage of EPSDT and transportation to and from medical providers (as per a recent regulation[8]), that might make them more generous than private health care insurance. The benchmark options include

- the Blue Cross/Blue Shield standard provider plan under the Federal Employees Health Benefits Program (FEHBP),
- a plan offered to state employees,
- the largest commercial health maintenance organization (HMO) in the state, and
- other Secretary-approved coverage appropriate for the targeted population.

Benchmark-equivalent coverage must have the same actuarial value as one of the benchmark plans identified above. Such coverage must include (1) inpatient and outpatient hospital services; (2) physician services; (3) lab and x-ray services; (4) emergency care; (5) well-child care, including immunizations; (6) prescribed drugs; (7) mental health services; and (8) other appropriate preventive care (designated by the Secretary). Such coverage must also include at least 75% of the actuarial value of coverage under the applicable benchmark plan for vision care and hearing services (if any).

For children under age 21 in one of the major mandatory and optional Medicaid eligibility groups, benchmark and benchmark-equivalent coverage must include EPSDT.

Also, Medicaid beneficiaries enrolled in such coverage must have access to services provided by rural health clinics and federally qualified health centers.

Starting in 2014, both benchmark and benchmark-equivalent packages must cover at least the essential health benefits that will also apply to plans in the private individual and small group health insurance markets. The 10 essential health benefits include (1) ambulatory patient services, (2) emergency services, (3) hospitalization, (4) maternity and newborn care, (5) mental health and substance use disorder services (including behavioral health treatment), (6) prescribed drugs, (7) rehabilitative and habilitative services and devices, (8) lab services, (9) preventive and wellness services and chronic disease management, and (10) pediatric services, including oral and vision care.[9] Many of these essential health benefits are currently coverable under benchmark packages. All benchmark plans must also cover family planning services and supplies.

Mental Health Parity Requirements Under Both Traditional Medicaid and Benchmark Plans

The federal mental health parity requirements, as established in the Public Health Service Act (Section 2726), generally require that, under a given insurance plan, coverage of mental health services (if offered) should be on par with coverage of medical and surgical services in terms of the treatment limitations (e.g., amount, duration and scope of benefits), financial requirements (e.g., beneficiary co-payments), in- and out-of-network covered benefits, and annual and lifetime dollar limits.

Managed care plans under both traditional Medicaid and benchmark packages must comply with all federal mental health parity requirements. Benchmark packages that are not managed care plans are only required to comply with federal requirements for parity in treatment limitations and financial requirements. However, these plans are deemed to comply with federal mental health parity requirements if they offer EPSDT, which they are statutorily required to cover.[10]

State Experience with Medicaid Benchmark Packages

As noted above, states have had the authority to implement benchmark benefit packages in their Medicaid programs since the Deficit Reduction Act of 2005.

A summary of state and territory experiences with benchmark benefits as of July 2012 is provided in *Table 4*. Of the 12 states and one territory (Guam) with approved benchmark plans, 11 had only one such plan and 2 (Idaho and Kentucky) had more than one benchmark plan. The type of benchmark used in 10 states and Guam was classified as secretary-approved, which generally means the benefit plan was tailored to the targeted population(s) to be enrolled.

Missouri had a plan classified as benchmark-equivalent to the FEHBP Blue Cross/Blue Shield standard option preferred provider organization (PPO). One of Kentucky's plans was identified as benchmark-equivalent to a state employee health plan, while Wisconsin provided coverage offered through the state's largest health maintenance organization (HMO), the United Health Care Choice Plus Plan.

In eight states (Connecticut, District of Columbia, Kansas, Minnesota, Missouri, Virginia, West Virginia, and Wisconsin) and Guam, benchmark plans were available statewide. In other states (Idaho, Kentucky, New York, and Washington), benchmark plans were limited to sub-state areas, such as specific counties or cities.

The state-level details with respect to the covered services offered through Medicaid benchmark plans were quite varied, at least in part reflecting the populations to be enrolled in these plans and the unique objectives of each state.

Preventive and primary care services (e.g., nutrition counseling, smoking cessation services, weight management counseling, dental care for adults) were covered in several states. Support services designed to facilitate independent living in community-based settings for individuals with disabilities and/or the elderly were components of benchmark plans in a few states.

There was also considerable state-level variation in other benchmark plan characteristics. Across the 17 state/plan combinations shown in *Table 4,*[11] there was almost an even split between benchmark programs for which enrollment was mandatory versus voluntary.

There was also quite a bit of variation in terms of the type of service delivery systems utilized. Fee-for-service alone (8 of 17 state/plan combinations) or in conjunction with some type of managed care arrangement (5 of 17 state/plan combinations) were the two most common service delivery system designs.

It is unclear how these state experiences to date with Medicaid benchmark plans will influence the design of such service packages roughly two years from now in 2014 when all states will be required to provide benchmark benefits to the new group of non-elderly, non-pregnant adults with income up to 133% of the federal poverty level. It is likely that states with no such experience will look to those states that have implemented benchmark packages for lessons learned in order to make choices tailored to their given circumstances and resources.

Table 4. Selected Characteristics of Medicaid Benchmark Plans

State and Eligibility Group(s)	Type of Benchmark	Examples of Covered Benefits	Enrollment Mandatory or Voluntary	Geographic Area	Delivery System
Connecticut; non-elderly, non-pregnant adults with income < 133% FPL	Secretary approved	Full state plan benefits under CT's traditional Medicaid program	Mandatory	Statewide	Fee-for-Service (FFS)
District of Columbia; non-elderly, non-pregnant adults with income < 133% FPL	Secretary approved	Standard Medicaid benefit package for adults (e.g., hospital care, MD services, Rx drugs, mental health care)	Mandatory	Statewide	Combination FFS and managed care
Guam; non-elderly, non-pregnant adults with income < 133% FPL	Secretary approved	Full state plan benefits as per Section 1905(a) of the Social Security Act	Mandatory	Statewide	FFS
Idaho-1; children and working age adults	Secretary approved	Standard Medicaid benefit package plus preventive care and nutrition services	Mandatory, with exceptions for changes in medical need	Statewide	Primary care case management (PCCM)
Idaho-2; individuals with disabilities or special health care needs and the elderly	Secretary approved	Preventive care, nutritional services and preventive health assistance plus all other Medicaid covered services	Voluntary (i.e., right to opt out and receive traditional Medicaid mandatory services)	Statewide	PCCM

Table 4. (Continued)

State and Eligibility Group(s)	Type of Benchmark	Examples of Covered Benefits	Enrollment Mandatory or Voluntary	Geographic Area	Delivery System
Idaho-3; elderly and persons dually eligible for Medicaid and Medicare	Secretary approved	All Medicaid covered services	Voluntary (i.e., right to opt out and receive traditional Medicaid mandatory services)	Select counties	Managed care (through Medicare Advantage Plans)
Kansas; certain working disabled populations	Secretary approved	State plan benefits plus independent living counseling to direct and manage needed services and budgets for that care; participants choose to self direct care or have an agency do so	Voluntary	Statewide	FFS with option to self direct care and use the cash and counseling model (e.g., purchase services of certain caregivers, such as a family member, that are provided in a home setting)
Kentucky-1; general Medicaid population; foster care and medically fragile children; elderly and disabled not opting into KY-3 and KY-4 (described below)	Secretary approved (Global Choices)	All mandatory benefits plus dental care; physical, occupational, speech therapy; non-emergency transportation, Rx drugs, prosthetic devices	Mandatory	Statewide (excluding 16 counties near Louisville operating under an 1115 waiver)	FFS
Kentucky-2; families	Benchmark-equivalent to state employee health plan	All mandatory benefits plus chiropractic services; speech,	Mandatory	Statewide (excluding 16 counties near Louisville operating	FFS

State and Eligibility Group(s)	Type of Benchmark	Examples of Covered Benefits	Enrollment Mandatory or Voluntary	Geographic Area	Delivery System
	(Family Choices)	physical and occupational therapy; home health and skilled nursing		under an 1115 waiver)	
Kentucky-3; individuals needing a nursing home level of care; includes such persons receiving care in the community	Secretary approved (Comprehensive Choices)	All mandatory benefits plus vision care, chiropractic services, dental care, hearing and audiometric services	Voluntary	Statewide (excluding 16 counties near Louisville operating under an 1115 waiver)	FFS
Kentucky-4; individuals with mental retardation and developmental disabilities who meet an ICF/MR level of care	Secretary approved (Optimum Choices)	All mandatory benefits plus dental care, vision care, chiropractic services, hearing and audiometric services	Voluntary	Statewide (excluding 16 counties near Louisville operating under an 1115 waiver)	FFS
Minnesota; non-elderly, non-disabled, non-pregnant adults otherwise ineligible for the state's traditional Medicaid and "prepaid medical assistance plus" programs with gross income < 75%	Secretary approved	Alcohol/drug treatment, chiropractic care, dental care, eyeglasses, family planning services, hospital services, interpreter services, home health care, nursing home and ICF-MR facility care,	Mandatory	Statewide	Combination FFS and managed care

Table 4. (Continued)

State and Eligibility Group(s)	Type of Benchmark	Examples of Covered Benefits	Enrollment Mandatory or Voluntary	Geographic Area	Delivery System
FPL (no resource test)		Prescriptions			
Missouri; parents and specified caretaker relatives up to 100% FPL—NOT IMPLEMENTED New York; categorically eligible adults ages 21 - 63	Benchmark equivalent to federal Blue Cross/Blue Shield Standard option preferred provider organization (PPO) Secretary approved	Selected traditional mandatory and optional benefits plus transplant related services Traditional state plan benefits plus medication therapy management	Mandatory Voluntary	Statewide Bronx	Combination FFS and managed care FFS
Virginia; certain working individuals with disabilities	Secretary approved	Traditional state plan benefits plus personal assistance services in various settings	Voluntary	Statewide	FFS
Washington; Aged, blind or disabled adults age 21+ with certain chronic, complex medical conditions (categorically needy only)	Secretary approved	Traditional state plan benefits plus chronic care management, coordination between behavioral health systems and other services (e.g., housing, transportation)	Voluntary	King County	Pre-paid ambulatory health plan and Regional Support Networks for mental health services
West Virginia; TANF and TANF-related individuals	Secretary approved	Basic package—all mandatory services plus home health,	Mandatory	Statewide	Combination managed care and FFS

State and Eligibility Group(s)	Type of Benchmark	Examples of Covered Benefits	Enrollment Mandatory or Voluntary	Geographic Area	Delivery System
		DME, prescribed drugs, tobacco cessation; Enhanced package—basic package plus weight management, podiatry, skilled nursing care, mental health care			
Wisconsin; pregnant women and infants with income between 200-250% FPL, and newborns of women with income between 200-250% FPL	State's largest HMO (United Health Care Choice Plus Plan)	Family planning, child health screenings, inpatient hospital services, mental health and substance abuse services, nursing home care, prescribed drugs, smoking cessation services, transportation	Mandatory	Statewide	Combination managed care, FFS, and PCCM

Source: Centers for Medicare & Medicaid Services, Office of Legislation, personal communication, July 26, 2012, based on information that was current as of July, 2012.

Notes: DME means durable medical equipment. ICF/MR means intermediate care facility for the mentally retarded that provides 24-hour rehabilitative and health care services for people with developmental disabilities. TANF refers to the Temporary Assistance for Needy Families program, which provides cash assistance to certain low-income families. PPO means preferred provider organization. Under the FFS delivery system, payments are made for each unit of service delivered. Under managed care delivery systems, payments are made on a predetermined, per-person-per-month basis. Under PCCM delivery systems, primary care physicians are paid a small, pre-set monthly fee per enrolled beneficiary to provide basic medical care, and serve as case managers or gate-keepers (via referrals) to specialty care (e.g., mental health care, dental services). A pre-paid ambulatory health plan provides less than comprehensive services on an at-risk or other than state plan reimbursement basis, and does not provide, arrange for, or otherwise have responsibility for the provision of any inpatient hospital or institutional services. Washington State had another Secretary-approved statewide benchmark plan similar to the plan outlined in this table in a single county. The King county-specific plan supersedes the statewide plan. Finally, New York state withdrew its program on June 7, 2012.

End Notes

[1] Beneficiary statistics for FY2011 were taken from Table 1.16, 2011 CMS Statistics, U.S. Department of Health and Human Services.

[2] Expenditure statistics for FY2010 were taken from Table III.2, 2011 CMS Statistics, U.S. Department of Health and Human Services.

[3] For example, pregnant women and children under age 6 with family income below 133% of FPL are mandatory eligibility groups under Medicaid. In 2012, the FPL for a family of four is $23,050—133% of FPL for a family of four would equal $30,656.50. See http://aspe.hhs.gov/poverty/12poverty.shtml.

[4] For a more detailed discussion, see the CRS Congressional Distribution Memo, Selected Issues Related to the Effect of NFIB v. Sebelius on the Medicaid Expansion Requirement in Section 2001 of the Affordable Care Act, by Kathleen S. Swendiman and Evelyne P. Baumrucker. Also see http://www.crs.gov/analysis/legalsidebar/pages/details.aspx?ProdId=117 and http://www.crs.gov/analysis/legalsidebar/pages/details.aspx?ProdId=121.

[5] For additional information about Section 1115 waivers, see CRS Report RL33202, Medicaid: A Primer.

[6] With respect to EPSDT, states also must provide medical care that is necessary to address health problems identified through screenings, including optional services that states may not otherwise cover in their Medicaid programs.

[7] These benchmark plans were later modified by the Children's Health Insurance Program Reauthorization Act of 2009 (P.L. 111-3) and the Patient Protection and Affordable Care Act (P.L. 111-148, as amended).

[8] Department of Health and Human Services, Centers for Medicare and Medicaid Services, Medicaid Program: States Flexibility for Medicaid Benefit Packages, Final Rule, 75 Federal Register, 23068 (April 30, 2010).

[9] See the "Essential Health Benefits Bulletin" at http://cciio.cms.gov/resources/files/Files2/12162011/ essential_health_benefits_bulletin.pdf. This document notes that CMS plans to issue further guidance on essential health benefits implementation in the Medicaid program.

[10] For more detailed information on mental health parity under Medicaid including substance use disorder services, see CRS Report R41768, Mental Health Parity and Mandated Coverage of Mental Health and Substance Use Disorder Services After the ACA, by Amanda K. Sarata.

[11] For additional details about Guam's Medicaid benchmark plan, see Table 4.

INDEX

E

F

G

H

I